the healing power of

REFLEXOLOGY

How the Restorative Power of Reflexology Can Help You Live a Balanced Life

Adams Media
New York London Toronto Sydney New Delhi

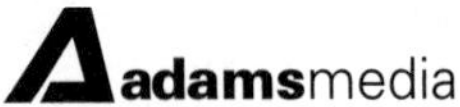

Adams Media
An Imprint of Simon & Schuster, Inc.
57 Littlefield Street
Avon, Massachusetts 02322

First Adams Media hardcover edition August 2019

For information about special discounts for bulk purchases, please contact Simon & Schuster Special Sales at 1-866-506-1949 or business@simonandschuster.com.

The Simon & Schuster Speakers Bureau can bring authors to your live event. For more information or to book an event contact the Simon & Schuster Speakers Bureau at 1-866-248-3049 or visit our website at www.simonspeakers.com.

Interior design by Stephanie Hannus
Interior images © 123RF/Kittikorn Phongok
Interior illustrations by Katelyn Rivera

Manufactured in the United States of America

10 9 8 7 6 5 4 3 2 1

Library of Congress Cataloging-in-Publication Data
Names: Adams Media, issuing body.
Title: The healing power of reflexology.
Description: Avon, Massachusetts: Adams Media, 2019.
Includes bibliographical references and index.
Identifiers: LCCN 2019006888 | ISBN 9781507210864 (hc) | ISBN 9781507210871 (ebook)
Subjects: LCSH: Reflexology (Therapy) | Self-care, Health.
Classification: LCC RM723.R43 H43 2019 | DDC 615.8/224--dc23
LC record available at https://lccn.loc.gov/2019006888

ISBN 978-1-5072-1086-4
ISBN 978-1-5072-1087-1 (ebook)

This book is intended as general information only, and should not be used to diagnose or treat any health condition. In light of the complex, individual, and specific nature of health problems, this book is not intended to replace professional medical advice. The ideas, procedures, and suggestions in this book are intended to supplement, not replace, the advice of a trained medical professional. Consult your physician before adopting any of the suggestions in this book, as well as about any condition that may require diagnosis or medical attention. The author and publisher disclaim any liability arising directly or indirectly from the use of this book.

Contains material adapted from the following title published by Adams Media, an Imprint of Simon & Schuster, Inc.: *Yoga Journal Presents Your Guide to Reflexology* by Yoga Journal, copyright © 2016, ISBN 978-1-4405-9381-9.

CONTENTS

INTRODUCTION

Heal your body, mind, and spirit with the ancient power of reflexology. Reflexology is an energetic touch therapy that works points on the feet (reflex points) that reflect specific areas of the body to promote deep relaxation and mindfulness. By opening yourself up to the wonders of reflexology, you can discover easy ways to enhance your life—or someone else's—with your own hands.

Reflexology is not linked to any one belief system. It can be practiced by anyone who is open to the healing power of touch. Whether you are healthy or are dealing with disease or injury, reflexology offers great benefits. When you are healthy, reflexology treatments can reinforce your vitality and strengthen your immune system; when ill, it can improve circulation, remove toxins, and stimulate the flow of energy throughout the body.

Extremely adaptable, reflexology also complements and supports other types of health treatments. People recovering from surgeries, cancer treatments, or any other severe conditions can benefit from reflexology sessions to promote healing. Also, reflexology sessions can easily be conducted in your home because you only need a comfortable chair for the recipient and a stool or chair for the giver.

The Healing Power of Reflexology presents reflexology not only as a healing art but also as a way to look at your life holistically. Reflexologists and other energy workers assist the receiver in focusing on the health of the body, mind, and spirit. In reflexology sessions, you can release troubling or busy thoughts, encourage muscles to let go of tension, and create an environment dedicated to whole wellness.

Reflexology can offer gentle yet powerful healing energies to you. All you have to do is open your heart to it and invite it in.

PART 1
What Is Reflexology?

Natural forces within us
are the true healers of disease.
—*HIPPOCRATES*

IN THIS PART, you'll discover what reflexology is (and isn't!). You'll take a step back to the past to look at the origins of reflexology around the world and trace its roots from the ancient Egyptian and Mayan cultures to the present day. You'll explore how the scientific revolution of the sixteenth century helped provide the intellectual framework for the practice of reflexology. And you'll look at how it is currently used.

Then you'll find out what reflexology can do for your body—it's not just for relieving stress; it is also useful for improving circulation, releasing toxins, and more. Curious about how reflexology can stimulate the body's own healing potential? This part will show you.

Finally, you'll take a tour of the human body as it relates to reflexology, looking at the structure and function of the body and how they are reflected in the feet. And don't worry, if you're unfamiliar with terms such as *zones*, *meridians*, and *chakras*, they are defined here—all with the intention of getting you ready to start healing!

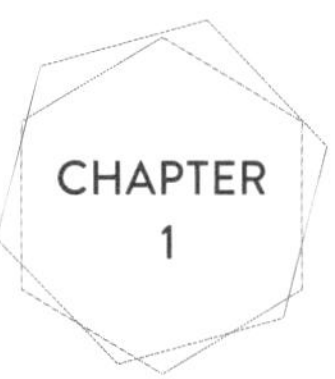

Reflexology Then and Now

To acquire knowledge, one must study;
but to acquire wisdom, one must observe.
—*MARILYN VOS SAVANT*

Taking a brief trip through the history of reflexology is a useful way to understand complementary, integrative healing approaches (also called modalities). Humans have left records that show an ancient tie to modern reflexology. Be they oral, artistic, or written, these accounts create a connection from the deep past to the clear present. In this chapter, you'll investigate those roots of reflexology, starting with ancient healing lore. Then you'll explore the scientific principles involved. Next you'll look at its evolution as it has grown in popularity throughout the twentieth and twenty-first centuries, up to the present day. Finally, you'll discover how professionals currently use reflexology. This grounding is intended to help you understand how reflexology and its fundamental techniques came about. But before we get to that, let's talk about what reflexology is and how it works.

What Is Reflexology?

Reflexology is an energetic touch therapy that works points on the feet (reflex points) that reflect specific areas of the body. If you imagine a body superimposed over the soles of the feet, you can begin to understand the basis of reflexology. The head is at the toes, and the rest of the body follows down the foot.

A reflexologist works with this concept, visualizing the areas that relate to the body as they are found on the feet. (In this book, we are limiting the discussion of reflexology to the feet; however, the hands are an important medium as well.)

The healing process is performed via a systematic application of pressure to reflex points using the thumbs and fingers. The technique is specific—certain thumb and finger movements are used to access the reflex points. The reflex points represent areas of the body itself, as well as organs and glands. The reflexing of these areas creates an overall feeling of euphoric relaxation.

Reflexologists work from the toes to the heels via a slow, gentle progression, reflexing the soles, the sides, and the tops of the feet. They also work points on the lower leg. As these areas are worked, the receiver begins to relax, experiencing the stress-relieving effects immediately. Often the recipient will feel a great sense of well-being flowing through the body. If the receiver has indicated a certain area of the body that is holding tension, the reflexologist will work both feet, returning to the areas mentioned by the recipient.

This modality creates a safe, trouble-free environment in which the receiver can release stress and find total relaxation. Reflexology helps teach the recipient the importance of letting go and provides the tool with which to accomplish this level of relaxation. A full session improves circulation; can create a sense of warmth; and promotes the elimination of toxins from the body, the restoration of peace of mind, and a deep sense of wholeness.

Ancient History

Many cultures use treating the feet as a way of healing the entire body. Its traces can be found throughout most ancient cultures, with references not only to working on the feet but also to the importance of feet in daily life and spiritual life.

Reflexology in Egypt

In Egypt, a pictograph in the tomb of Ankhmahor, who was the physician to the king at Saqqara, shows an early example of reflexology. The section of the picture dealing with reflexology portrays two physicians working. One doctor is holding a foot, the other is holding a hand, and both are attending to these extremities. Clearly Egypt is a strong root in the history tree of reflexology.

• • • Reflex Points • • •

During the process of mummification in ancient Egypt, the soles of the feet were removed to free the soul to travel beyond the earthly plane. In fact, many ancient cultures believed the feet were a key to the higher being, the sole-to-soul connection.

Throughout the World

The ancient Egyptian world wasn't the only one that practiced a form of reflexology. In China, writings as old as the fourth century B.C. speak of a therapy where pressure is applied by the fingers to the feet, hands, and ears. Eventually, this therapy evolved to the use of needles (acupuncture) along energy lines called meridians. However, pressure from the thumbs and fingers continued to be used as well.

Shogo Mochizuki, author and educator, tells us that in Japan you can hear the proverb "The foot is the gate of ten thousand different illnesses." This proverb illustrates the journey of reflexology. The ancient art was carried over from China and continued by healers in Japan.

In India, the feet of Buddha and the feet of Vishnu both have symbols representing life and the flow of energy to live life well. The symbols are not reflex points, but they do seem to be placed in areas on the feet where a reflexologist might work.

The Bible also mentions feet as a way of healing. To wash the feet of another was a symbol of humility and forgiveness. To remove shoes before entering the temple or holy place is an instruction found in the Bible, and is also a practice followed by Buddhists, Muslims, and Hindus.

Pre-Columbian and Native American Lore

You may be wondering whether reflexology was practiced on the other side of the world. Some people believe that the Incan people were the first Americans to practice reflexology, but no concrete evidence of this exists. However, it is thought that the ancient Mayan civilization shows documentation of reflexology. The altar at Copán, Honduras, has engravings of a Mayan reflexology treatment, according to reflexologist Jürgen Kaiser, revealing a clear connection between reflexology and the Mayan culture.

• • • Reflex Points • • •

Reference to the use of reflexology is found in most eras. In every class of people, from medical practice to home remedy, reflexology has held a place of importance. Practitioners of reflexology feel this is a unique form of work that can help anyone and can never cause harm if done correctly.

Native American cultures speak through oral history of the tradition of bathing and treating the feet to help bring about balance. The history of these cultures demonstrates many natural healing techniques, of which most are still used today. These are just a few examples of how footwork has been in the Americas for a long time!

As you can see, reflexology has crossed all boundaries, both cultural and geographical. We have been able to trace the physical and spiritual connections of reflexology to the past, but what about the scientific connections?

Scientific Roots

Reflexology finds its scientific roots in a form of pressure therapy that was practiced in Europe during the 1500s. The term *reflex* first appeared in the field of physiology in 1771. Further research in movement resulted in the concept of "reflex action," which everyone is now familiar with. Thank goodness for reflex action, or we would step on that tack!

From England and France to Germany and Russia, research from the late 1800s through the twentieth century produced extraordinary theories and hypotheses. Much of that work is useful in the understanding of reflexology. For instance, neurological studies connecting the brain and the entire nervous system illustrated how nerve endings in the feet could create a dialogue with the entire body, and how, conversely, stimulation of an organ can cause movement in the feet.

The Twentieth Century

The precursor to modern reflexology, zone therapy, was brought to the US by Dr. William Fitzgerald. In the early twentieth century, he worked in London and then Vienna, where zone therapy was in use. When he returned to the US, he began to talk about zone therapy, encouraging others in the medical field to learn this drug-free modality. While Fitzgerald was influenced by what he saw and read while in Europe, he developed his own theories regarding zone therapy and reflexes.

Fitzgerald began to record the areas of pain, the conditions that caused the pain, and the resulting relief. He experimented with various areas of the body and charted his findings. He divided the body into ten zones. Each zone runs from a toe up to the head and out to a finger and back again, separating the body into ten parts. Any place on a zone can be affected by pressing points on the feet and/or hands. For instance, Fitzgerald found that if you have a headache, you can press your great toe (your big toe) or your thumb to help relieve the pain.

••• Reflex Points •••

Dr. Fitzgerald's zones are different from—but similar to—the meridians mentioned earlier. Meridians, which come from traditional Chinese medicine, are the twelve energy lines that run through the body, either beginning or ending in the feet or hands.

Influencing Others

Fitzgerald learned through his research and practical application how to relieve painful symptoms, often without anesthesia. He published a book, *Zone Therapy*, in 1917 and lectured and demonstrated his findings to his colleagues. Some accepted his findings, though many did not. Even some doctors who did find zone therapy effective felt the practice was too unorthodox and time-consuming to adopt. However, some dentists, chiropractors, naturopaths, and others in the medical field preferred a drugless treatment and began to use the zone method.

One doctor who believed in the practice of zone therapy was Dr. Joe Shelby Riley. Together with his wife, he operated a school in Washington, DC, covering many drug-free therapies. Riley did not use any of the tools that Dr. Fitzgerald had employed; rather, he created a technique using his fingers and thumbs. He spent time documenting in charts the regions he felt were affected within the zones.

The Mother of Reflexology

Dr. Fitzgerald and Dr. Riley may have introduced this concept in the US, but a third person was responsible for truly introducing reflexology to the modern world. Eunice Ingham, a therapist working for Dr. Riley in the 1930s, accepted zone therapy completely. Ingham is considered the mother of reflexology and is honored by all reflexologists. Through her work with Dr. Riley, Ingham moved zone therapy into a new modality she called reflexology. Ingham saw a correlation between glands and points in the feet, and she felt that working these points was key to zone pressure therapy.

• • • Reflex Points • • •

Ingham connected the actual anatomy of the body with the zones. She introduced the concept of the feet as a mirror image of the body structure. Ingham's belief that the sensitivity of the feet improved the treatment led reflexologists to ignore hands as a medium for many years. We now know that both hands and feet are effective in enhancing reflexology treatment.

In Ingham's book *Stories the Feet Have Told Thru Reflexology*, published in 1951, she introduces the importance of nerves in the feet. She explains that her method, the Ingham Compression Method of Reflexology, can help alleviate congestion in certain areas of the body, particularly in the glandular system. Ingham separated reflexology from zone therapy and recognized this as a new modality, further removing the treatment from massage. Equally as important, Ingham continued a dialogue with the medical community, holistic practitioners, and the lay consumer.

Reflexology Today

Reflexologists continued to practice Ingham's self-help treatment, and the method is still taught in her school, the International Institute of Reflexology, located in St. Petersburg, Florida. Many renowned authors and reflexologists have studied this method, and it is widely recognized as the root of modern reflexology.

Today, a national testing board administers a voluntary exam that further certifies a professional reflexologist. This board encourages continuing education and provides a referral service to consumers of nationally certified reflexologists.

Reflexology has come a long way over the course of human history! Integrative health practice is an essential part of healing today. Many reputable reflexology schools around the world prepare professional practitioners in this field. There are professional associations worldwide; we even celebrate World Reflexology Week in September. Teaching conferences are held annually in various countries and states. You can even find apps related to reflexology for your smartphone!

• • • Reflex Points • • •

As you read this book and practice reflexology on yourself, your friends, and your family, do not use reflexology in lieu of a medical consultation. If you or someone you perform reflexology on is under a doctor's care, make sure to work within the guidelines set by the doctor.

Current Applications

Chronic stress is the cause of many debilitating diseases. This knowledge allows the practice of reflexology to come to the forefront of treatment, as reflexology reduces stress and promotes whole health. The recognition of reflexology as a true integrative health treatment has begun in earnest: the field of cancer research is using reflexology, as is holistic nursing. Hospitals employ reflexologists in many capacities. Doctors are sending their staff to become trained reflexologists. Hospice is beginning to use the compassionate touch of reflexology.

As reflexology is recognized for the viable healing modality that it is, the research into it will only expand. In the meantime, you can learn how reflexology works and how to do a session on your family and friends. You can help people become less stressed, and you can help yourself feel great too!

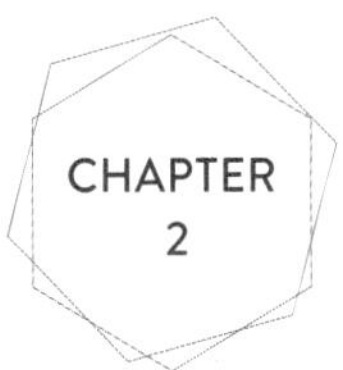

CHAPTER 2

What Reflexology Can Do

Health is a state of complete harmony of the body, mind, and spirit. When one is free from physical disabilities and mental distractions, the gates of the soul open.

—B.K.S. IYENGAR

It's amazing what reflexology can actually do! Consistent, uniform sessions of reflexology create a receptive environment for whole health. The message to relax and to let the body function properly is relayed with every session. The body, mind, and spirit respond to this technique, allowing for overall self-improvement and healing to occur.

In this chapter, you'll explore how reflexology can reduce stress, improve circulation, release toxins, and stimulate your body's ability to heal itself. The chapter also discusses how the regular practice of reflexology can help balance the energy flow through your body. Finally, you'll be shown how reflexology can assist in maintaining your overall health. By the end of the chapter, you won't be asking, "What can reflexology do?" you'll be asking, "What *can't* it do?"

Reduce Stress

Stress is part of life. Without stressors we would have no challenge, no stimulation—what would excite us? To be alive is to experience stress. Some people function well under crisis, while others do not. How people adapt to stress dictates the effect the stressor has on them.

Each time a person overreacts to the experience of a negative stress factor, the proper flow of energy throughout the body is disrupted. Ultimately the body's systems may become too congested and begin to shut down, causing a break somewhere in the proper function of the miraculous body.

• • • Reflex Points • • •

Stress is a very real physiological reaction. Undue stress causes a rapid release of hormones into the bloodstream as the body prepares to use more energy. To be constantly "on" is what produces chronic stress. Many people do not know how to slow down.

Carrying an overabundance of stress may invite such developments as chronic fatigue, headaches, teeth grinding, and excessive anger. Chronic muscle fatigue is another side effect of stress overload. Excessive stress may cause anxiety and depression as well as a weakened immune system. Heart disease and cancer have also been linked to constant stress.

How you respond to stress is a key factor that determines your wellness. Some people are able to go through the day without overreacting to everyday stressors, while others cannot cope as well. Any negative responses generated from stress may weaken your body's systems, leaving you open to future complications.

Balance the Energy Flow in the Body

When your body is functioning at its optimum, you are in a state of homeostasis, which means balance. With homeostasis, every system of your body is working properly; you are a fine-tuned machine, running at full production. The central nervous system, which consists of the brain and spinal cord, sends messages through the nerves directing every part of your being to act properly. This basic operating function happens without any outside stimulus.

Energy flows through the body by way of electrical impulses and chemical messengers such as hormones or endorphins. How does that work? Some pathways of energy move with the nervous system, and others use meridians, zones, chakras, or, simply put, the universal life force.

• • • Reflex Points • • •

There are ten zones, twelve main meridians, and seven main chakras, all of which divide the body into sections. Each of these sections is connected to the structure, function, and well-being of the body and can be accessed through reflexology.

What Is This Energy?

The energy we are talking about here is the shared energy that makes up everything on this planet. Humans connect into this universal energy through their own energy fields. The body's energy fields are composed of many electrical functions dispersed throughout the organic systems. You have electrochemical, electromagnetic, and many other electrical impulses working to maintain balance in your body. The molecules of the body run through many pathways of energy, balancing your systems in a continuous cycle.

• • • Reflex Points • • •

"Universal life force energy" has many names throughout the world's cultures, such as chi, qi, ki, prana, Shakti, Reiki, spirit, yesod, waken, baraka, and orenda. You have probably heard at least one or two of these names before.

Congestion and Blockages of Energy

Energy can become congested or blocked, and stimulation through reflexology may break up this interference, allowing energy to once again flow freely throughout the body. An area becomes blocked or congested when the body overloads with toxins. Toxins are any substances that interfere with homeostasis, interrupting the smooth flow of body function.

Some of these congested areas may be actual stressed regions found in the feet. Scar tissue from a past injury, calluses, or pinched nerves, as well as a buildup of uric acid can all be the cause of blockages. Other causes may be emotional upsets, which can produce an overall feeling of listlessness and exhaustion. Emotional stress can bring about muscle tension, headaches, and even an upset stomach. The extended blockage of energy channels can result in long-term illness or pain. Chronic pains, which may manifest as fibromyalgia, myofascial pain syndrome, arthritis, or irritable bowel syndrome, are clear examples of energy disruption. When a reflex feels tight, this reflects as a congestion of an energy pathway.

Improve Circulation

Have you ever noticed your feet when you have been sitting for a very long time, perhaps on a transatlantic air flight or a cross-country drive? They may look puffy, swollen, or discolored, because the circulation of blood in your body hasn't been energized for a while. In other words, you didn't move around a lot. Poor circulation can occur for many reasons. Reflexology is a powerful adjunct for improving circulation, along with whatever has been prescribed medically.

Blood circulates to every cell in the body through an intricate system that contains more than 60,000 miles of blood vessels. Reflexology encourages oxygen, blood, and lymph to move through the body, assisting in proper circulation.

Regular sessions of reflexology help chronic circulatory issues. A receiver who has diabetes, has Raynaud's phenomenon, smokes, or is on a medication that may affect circulation could benefit from reflexology. In any of these cases, a series of eight weekly sessions can bring about noticeable improvements. Following that, continued monthly sessions can help to maintain enhanced circulation.

Release Toxins

Picture oxygenated blood traveling through the arteries of your body, the rich blood nourishing you. Some of that blood travels down until it eventually reaches the feet. Here the law of gravity kicks in, and many of the toxins that the blood may have picked up are dropped off in the feet, before the veins begin the process of carrying the oxygen-stripped blood back up to be recharged. Reflexology helps with the removal of these toxic wastes by revving up the body to work smoothly and efficiently so that it flushes out waste material. The removal comes through some form of excretion (sweat, urine, and bowel movements) as the body works to rid itself of any unfriendly substances.

The lymphatic system is another waste-removing component within our bodies. The lymph vessels and organs deal with the absorption of fats, the distribution of excess fluids, and the elimination of other harmful substances. Reflexology helps to support the work of the lymph and spleen, thus encouraging the lymphatic movement throughout the body.

Stimulate the Body's Own Healing Potential

By now you can see that our bodies are very smart! Sometimes they may need a little push (on the feet) to get them working correctly, but they can pretty much take care of themselves. Reflexology is the gentle guide to remind the body to wake up and do what it should be doing. Every system of the body needs to work in unison with the others. Bones without muscles would fall on the floor, and blood without oxygen couldn't feed the body, just as food couldn't turn into energy without digestion and elimination.

Whole Health

Whole health is what you are capable of producing for yourself by proactively being involved with your body. Reflexology affects every system of the body, paving the way for whole healing. The immune system protects the body from external organisms. The body works to recognize, eliminate, and resist all outside influences that detract from homeostasis. This modality encourages the immune system to continually defend the body from all toxic invasions.

Prevention through a healthful lifestyle is a natural way to reach your highest potential. Reflexology—along with good eating habits, exercise, and positive thinking—can help you stay healthy. What you believe you are—you are! Picture yourself as happy and healthy, and go for it.

Assist in Maintaining a State of Health

If you're healthy, reflexology will support your continued good health. Reflexology gives a jump-start to a healthier lifestyle when needed. If you know someone who could use some positive reinforcement and support, reflexology is a great tool for doing so. Reflexology can enable people to relax and let go of what ails them, at least for the time they are experiencing treatment. The resulting sense of well-being can help them feel in charge of their health and move forward on the path of improved wellness.

The more reflexology treatment a person receives, the better that person will feel. Subtle changes will begin to take place within the internal balance. Reflexology also complements and supports any existing medical treatments. As a healing art, reflexology encourages healing from within. The body works with the innate intelligence of your mind and the spiritual wisdom of your soul in developing whole health.

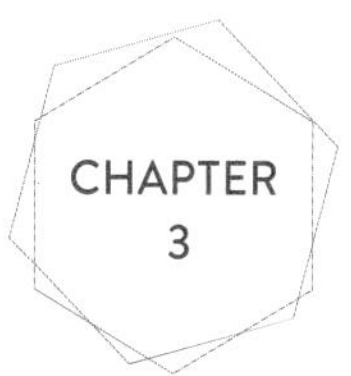

CHAPTER 3

Understanding the Body As It Relates to Reflexology

If you're feeling out of kilter, don't know why or what about, let your feet reveal the answer, find the sore spot, work it out.

—EUNICE INGHAM

Reflexology is based on the premise that the feet and hands are a microcosm of the body—that the parts reflect the whole. Imagine a tiny body superimposed over the feet, with the toes as its head. Every aspect of the body is reflected on the feet—every bone, muscle, nerve, blood vessel, and organ. Manipulating the feet, then, is a way to manipulate these areas.

In this chapter, you'll learn how reflexology connects with the different parts of the body. You'll investigate both the structure and function of the body, and how these are represented in the feet. You'll also get a little more in-depth information about zones, meridians, and chakras. In the end, you'll have a clearer understanding of the body as it is seen through the lens of reflexology.

The Structure of the Body

The anatomical structure of the body is the organization of the various components of the body and the relationship between the levels of this organization. Cells (one component) are organized into tissues. Tissues are organized into organs, and organs are organized into organ systems. Let's take a more in-depth look at this organization.

Chemicals combine to create the cells that form the structure of all living organisms. Each cell metabolizes, breathes, reproduces, and excretes. Metabolism is the interaction of all the chemicals that pass through a cell. Metabolism is continuous. Food is taken in and then used in whatever part of the cell structure it is needed. After the food is processed, the waste is eliminated and the process begins again.

The Tissue

Cell groups that have the same structure and function form tissue. The human body has four major types of tissue. These categories are epithelial, connective, muscle, and nervous tissue. Each of these groups performs a particular function. Epithelial tissue covers the body and lines the organs. Connective tissue basically provides support and protection to the body. Muscle tissue allows movement. Nervous tissue is a major component of the nervous system, which has the ability to receive and send signals.

The Organs

The next level of structural organization is formed when tissues group together to become organs. Organs are structures with specific functions. As the organs group together in related function, they form systems. These body systems work in concert to produce a complete living entity, an organism.

The anatomical regions that contain the internal organs are known as body cavities. Knowledge of these areas is helpful in explaining the position of many of the reflexes. There are two main cavities. One is the cavity found on the back of the body, and the other is found in the front. The back region is divided into two parts—one holds the brain and the other the spinal cord. The front cavity is also divided into two parts—the chest region and the abdominopelvic region. The two divisions of the frontal cavity contain all the major organs of the body. These divisions help us to picture the body superimposed over the foot as we locate the reflexes associated with these areas.

The Function of the Body

Each organ system performs a specific function. However, organ systems need to work together to survive. The cooperative relationship between the systems presents the highest level of organization within the body.

The eleven major organ systems of the body are:

1. Integumentary—the skin and related structures
2. Skeletal—bones, cartilages, and joints
3. Muscular—muscle tissue
4. Nervous—brain, spinal cord, nerves, and sense organs
5. Endocrine—all the glands that produce hormones
6. Respiratory—lungs and all air passageways
7. Cardiovascular—blood, heart, and blood vessels
8. Lymphatic—lymph, lymph vessels, and lymph structures
9. Digestive—teeth, esophagus, stomach, and associated glands
10. Urinary—kidney, bladder, and related ducts
11. Reproduction—ovaries, testes, and all reproductive structures

The Integumentary System

The integumentary system is primarily the skin, and it provides a protective covering over the entire body. Skin regulates the temperature of the body, metabolizes nutrients from the sun, and excretes waste through sweat. Skin is a receptor for stimuli from the environment and communicates this information to the nervous system. Reflexology is a powerful stimulus that works to support the efforts of the integumentary system.

The Skeletal System

The skeletal system is composed of all the bones, joints, and cartilages of the body. The skeleton contains 206 bones that are attached by ligaments, tendons, and muscles. Bones provide support for motion and leverage, as well as protection for the body and its organs. Bones also store minerals and produce blood cells. Reflexology may increase blood circulation, which in turn nourishes skeletal cells. It can also aid in healing surrounding areas in the event of a bone fracture.

The Muscular System

Although bones provide leverage and make up the frame of the body, they cannot move by themselves. The muscular system provides the movement necessary for the body through the contraction and relaxation of muscles. Contracting muscles create motion, maintain posture, and produce heat.

Muscles that move voluntarily can contract by the use of your conscious mind. Walking, running, talking, or any conscious intent of motion is performed by the voluntary use of skeletal muscles. You can decide to move out of your seat to greet a friend, for example, or to shake hands upon an introduction.

• • • Reflex Points • • •

As you walk, you affect your entire body. Every feeling–good, bad, or indifferent–emanates from the feet. The way you walk dictates how the entire body functions. Proper gait allows for good posture and a pain-free existence. Many aches and pains in the body can be directly related to the feet.

Cardiac muscles and smooth muscles take direction only from certain systems and are not controlled by your conscious mind. You can hold your breath until you pass out, for example, but then the smooth muscles will take over in response to the lack of oxygen, meaning that your lungs will start to work again.

The muscular system may become taxed from simple activities such as sitting at your desk for long hours, lifting heavy objects, or even emotional strain manifesting in tense or tight muscles. When muscles are tense, the body's energy is imbalanced. Reflexology stimulates nerve endings in the feet to release energy, which in turn promotes increased muscle relaxation.

The Nervous System

The activities of the body are regulated through this system. This structure detects and responds to changes in the internal and external environments. The nervous system has two major divisions: the central nervous system (CNS), which is the brain and spinal cord, and the peripheral nervous system (PNS), which is composed of the spinal and cranial nerves.

• • • Reflex Points • • •

The nervous system is like a computer. The brain is the mainframe. The nerves are the connecting wires that reach out through the body to all the systems that are connected to the brain. Sensory nerves send messages from the body systems to the brain, and motor nerves send the brain's response back to the body.

The nervous system keeps communication active between all systems in the body. Reflexology works with the 7,200 nerve endings in the feet, affecting the nervous system and all related areas.

The Endocrine System

The endocrine system controls and integrates body functions through hormones that are secreted into the bloodstream. The endocrine system—together with the central nervous system—holds the primary responsibility of controlling the complex activities of the body. Both are communication networks. The central nervous system transmits its messages through electrochemical impulses while the endocrine system employs chemical messengers in the form of hormones released into the bloodstream.

Hormones affect the body in four basic ways:

1. They control the internal environment of the body.
2. They help the body cope with emergencies.
3. They assist in growth and development.
4. They aid in the process of reproduction.

All hormones are essential in the maintenance of homeostasis, as they alter cell activity to promote balance. The body controls the production of these chemicals, producing only what is necessary. Reflex points relate to the hormone-producing glands; reflexology helps to maintain the desired balance.

The Respiratory System

This system supplies oxygen to the blood and eliminates carbon dioxide. The respiratory system carries air in and out of the lungs. The process of respiration involves three procedures. The first step is breathing, the act of exchanging air between the lungs and the atmosphere. The other two steps, known as external and internal respiration, involve the exchange of gases between the lungs and the blood, and then the exchange of gases between the blood and the cells. Reflexology helps to create a healthy environment for breathing, especially when the giver provides the receiver with constant reminders to relax and breathe.

The Cardiovascular System

The cardiovascular system transports respiratory gases, nutrients, wastes, and hormones. This system protects against disease and fluid loss, and regulates body temperature and acid-base balance. The cardiovascular system not only provides nourishment and life to all parts of the body; it also transports energy for thought and action.

The heart is built to pump large quantities of blood and push it through the vessels throughout the body so that the exchange of oxygen and carbon dioxide can occur. Arteries carry oxygen-rich blood out of the heart into the body, and veins bring the depleted blood back to the heart. Working together, the lungs and heart move the blood in a continuous, ceaseless circle.

Reflexology promotes circulation, augmenting the work of the cardiovascular system and supporting the heart and the vessels.

The Lymphatic System

Lymph vessels and organs work with the cardiovascular system to transport food and oxygen to the tissues of the body. Both systems remove waste as well. However, the lymph system moves in only one direction, toward the heart. The fluid recovered from the tissues, known as lymph, is returned to the circulatory structure to be used again. The lymph nodes filter out toxins before the fluid reaches the blood for reuse. Reflexology works to keep the pathways clear, allowing for smooth transition of lymph.

The Digestive System

The digestive system begins with food entering the mouth. The food is conducted down through the body, nutrients are removed from it, and then the waste is eliminated. Many organs are involved with the function of digesting and eliminating. This system works by breaking down food, absorbing nutritional substances into the body, and then converting them into yet other substances that replenish and refuel the cells. This is a process that gives us vitality, strength, and continued growth.

Reflexology works to bring about homeostasis for each organ within the digestive system, assisting in the overall proper function of these structures.

The Urinary System

The urinary system removes toxins from the blood and maintains the acid-base balance of the body. This system regulates the chemical composition, volume, and electrolyte balance of the blood. The urinary system works in conjunction with the respiratory, integumentary, and digestive organs to eliminate waste. The excretory organs of these systems offer other avenues for the waste products of metabolism to be released. A primary function of reflexology is to remove toxins and help to reestablish harmony. Reflexology supports and enhances the urinary system.

• • • Reflex Points • • •

All of the body systems work together to produce homeostasis. All systems interact; none can exist without the whole. Reflexology treats the whole person and supports the work of the body in its entirety.

The Reproductive System

Male and female reproductive systems have different organs, although their functions from the perspective of reflexology are basically the same. Reproduction is procreation, the continuation of our species, the sustaining of human life. This miraculous process not only reproduces cells; it also allows genetic material to live on through the generations.

Some points on the feet are associated with the reproductive areas, and manipulating those spots through reflexology can help to address some of the imbalances that affect fertility.

The Body Is Mirrored in the Feet

The feet are tiny mirrors of the body. Each and every part of the body is replicated on the feet.

- The right foot contains all of the right side of the body, back and front.
- The left foot holds the left side of the body, back and front.
- The tops of the feet are representative of the back of the body, and the soles of the feet symbolize the front of the body.
- The inside arch areas of the feet represent the spine.
- The outer edges and sides of the feet denote the outer edges of the body, from the head to the feet.

The feet tell many stories about the people they are connected to. The color and temperature are important indicators of a person's state of well-being. How the feet are cared for is a sign of how the person cares for herself or himself. Congestion, pain, swelling, discomfort, or discoloration on the feet is representative of some stressful element in the body. Whatever the cause, the reflexologist will gently work the area to relieve the receiver's discomforts, if possible. The giver works with the intention to release stress and promote relaxation.

• • • Reflex Points • • •

The temptation to diagnose a condition may arise when performing reflexology. Do not give in! Reflexology fights stress and makes people feel better. Reflexology does not cure. Reflexologists do not prescribe medical treatments; they refer people back to their doctors for the treatment of a condition.

Understanding where the body is represented on the feet gives you a deeper understanding of what may be affecting the person you are working on. Feet have a story to tell.

Zones

Do you remember Dr. Fitzgerald from Chapter 1? He was the doctor who introduced zone therapy to the US. Fitzgerald worked and researched in Europe where the concept of zone therapy was evolving. He worked with the theory of longitudinal zones dividing the body. According to this theory, the body has ten zones that run from the head to the feet, as shown in Figure 3.1

Every organ and body part in a zone can be affected by applying pressure to the feet and hands. An imaginary separation occurs at the centerline of the body, with five zones on the right side and five zones on the left.

The vertical zones guide us to work with each toe or finger so that we touch the entire zone within that energy field. If a blockage or congestion exists anywhere along a line in that zone, pressure applied to the corresponding reflex will help clear it. Often pain or discomfort manifesting in one area of a zone may actually be a referral from somewhere else along that zone.

Transverse zones are divided by imaginary horizontal lines that separate the feet into four sections. These areas are:

- The shoulder line, located under the necks of the toes.
- The diaphragm line, tucked under the ball of the foot.
- The waistline, found in the middle of the arch.
- The sciatic line, situated across the center of the heel.

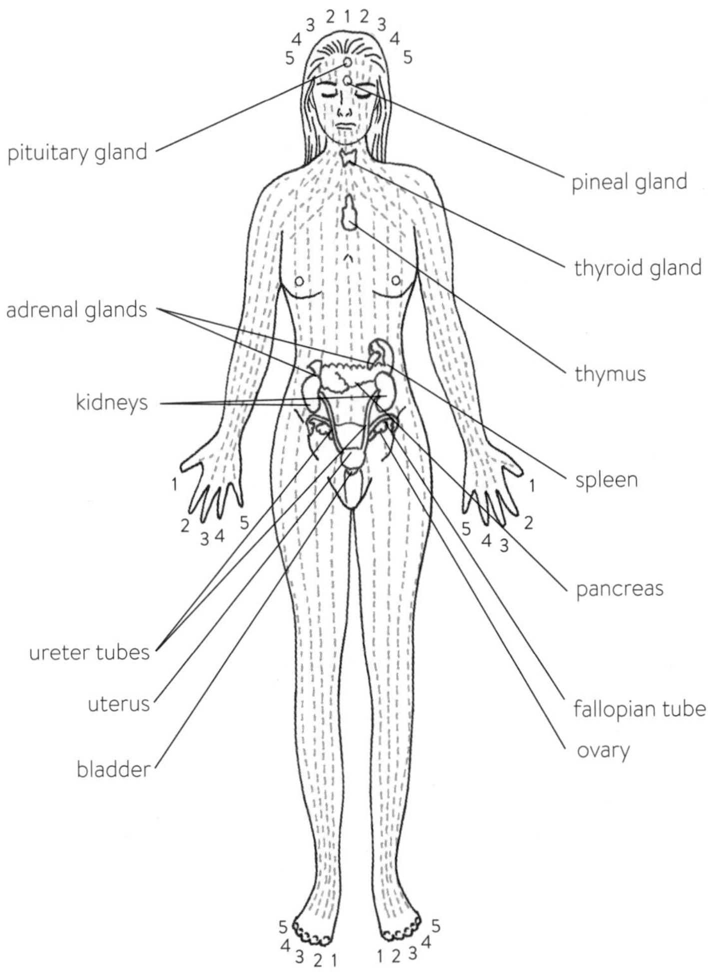

Figure 3.1 The body is divided into ten longitudinal zones.

Meridians

Traditional Asian medicine looks to balance chi or ki (life force or energy) and to keep it flowing through the energy channels called meridians. Reflexology and acupuncture are two modalities that focus their work around the concept of energy channels. Both believe that by manipulating these channels, blockages that could cause disease can be prevented. While acupuncture points are found all over the body, reflexology points are on the feet and reflected on the hands. By using pressure that disperses congestion along the energy pathways, the energy can flow freely, encouraging wellness.

• • • Reflex Points • • •

Meridians are also found in other healing systems such as shiatsu and acupressure.

The meridians run vertically through the body, beginning or ending in either the hands or feet. Reflexology affects the meridians; many of the reflexes are actually on meridian lines. These energetic pathways connect with the systems of the body. An obstruction along a meridian may disrupt the function of organs found on that channel. Six standard meridians run on the legs—three yin (earth energy) and three yang (sun energy). Six more run on the arms using the same divisions. The energy of all meridians moves continuously in a steady flow.

Foot reflexology works with the six standard meridians that run on the legs. Each is connected to a specific organ.

The Twelve Standard Meridians and the Two Vessels

Energy follows pathways that run through both sides of the body. The two vessels that are most often used with the twelve meridians run along the middle line of the body, in the front and the back. These two vessels divide the body and balance the meridians. The twelve standard meridians and the two vessels are as follows:

- Lung meridian
- Large intestine meridian
- Stomach meridian
- Spleen/pancreas meridian
- Heart meridian
- Small intestine meridian
- Bladder meridian
- Kidney meridian
- Circulatory/pericardium meridian
- Endocrine meridian
- Gallbladder meridian
- Liver meridian
- Conception vessel
- Governing vessel

The Six Meridians of the Feet

The six meridians represented in the feet, specifically in the toes, are the spleen/pancreas, stomach, kidney, bladder, liver, and gallbladder.

- **The spleen/pancreas meridian**, which works in partnership with the stomach meridian, starts at the tip of the great toe, runs up the leg, turns in at the pelvis, goes up the side of the abdomen, and ends in the shoulder.
- **The stomach meridian** starts under the eye, curves along the face and up to the temple, then continues down the body and ends on top of the second toe. Many believe the stomach to be one of the root causes of upsets throughout the body. The stomach meridian is the channel that actually touches all the major organs. Stomach problems are often reflected elsewhere in the body.
- **The kidney meridian** begins on the sole directly in the solar plexus reflex in the center of the foot beneath the ball. The path runs along the inside of the leg and thigh up to the bladder area, past the navel and breastbone, and ending on the

sternum side of the clavicle. Changes in this meridian can indicate kidney and/or circulation irregularities.

- **The bladder meridian** starts at the inner corner of the eye and runs up and over the skull, dividing into two strands at the back of the neck. The strands run down as parallel lines along the entire back to the coccyx (tailbone) area. From the coccyx, one strand of the pathway continues through to the heel and ends on the little toe. The other strand ends in the hollow of the knee. Changes in this meridian may denote painful conditions such as headaches, rheumatic pains, sciatica, and eczema.
- **The liver meridian** starts between the first and second toe, runs along the inside of the leg, past the groin and bladder, touches the ribs, and ends in the chest. Changes in this meridian may be indicated by jaundice, fatigue, swelling of the liver, intestinal disorders, allergies, and headaches.
- **The gallbladder meridian** is the last of the meridians in the feet. This meridian begins at the outer eye and runs through the temple to the back, then down to the top of the pelvis and along the outside of the leg to the fourth toe. Congestion along this meridian may be associated with acute and chronic pain. The disorders affiliated with the gallbladder pathway are migraines, teeth and ear pain, jaw pain, pain in the lower limbs, and neuralgia.

• • • Reflex Points • • •

Meridians and reflexes often cross paths. Reflexology includes the stimulation of points along meridian lines. These two ways of understanding the body (zones and meridians) complement each other and can help givers and receivers better understand problem areas that have manifested on the feet.

Chakras

Chakra is a Sanskrit word meaning "wheel." This concept of energy focuses on energy wheels that spin at key positions within the body. Chakras deal with the expression of energy in our physical, emotional, mental, and spiritual essence.

The human energy system flows freely with the help of the chakras. Chakras balance and distribute life force energy to create homeostasis among all systems and functions within the body. Congestion of the body can cause these wheels to become blocked, meaning that they operate at less than optimum potential. Chakras and meridians share many connections. These vital energy centers influence our whole being.

Location of the Major Chakras

The root, or base, chakra is the first wheel and is located at the coccyx, the tailbone of the spine. The gonads, which are the ovaries and testes, are the glands connecting this chakra with the endocrine system. The areas of the body affected are the lower extremities, legs and feet, and also the skeletal system, large intestine, and spine. The nervous system is also connected with the root chakra. The root chakra deals with the issues of survival and security, connecting us with our family and our profession.

The sacral chakra, the second wheel, is found at the sacrum. The organs affiliated with this chakra are the reproductive organs, the kidneys, and the bladder. The circulatory system and the lymphatic system are linked as well. The adrenal glands are the connection to the endocrine system. The sacral chakra connects with our awareness of abundance, sensuality, and sexuality.

The solar plexus (center) chakra, the third wheel, is located in the center of the body. The respiratory system, stomach, gallbladder, and liver are the functions of the body connected to this chakra. The pancreas represents the link to the endocrine system. The solar plexus center deals with our sense of self, connecting us with our sense of empowerment.

The heart chakra, the fourth wheel, is directly related to the physical heart. The respiratory, circulatory, and immune systems are connected with this center, as well as the arms and hands. The heart chakra is our emotional center, responding to our feelings of love and joy.

The throat chakra, the fifth wheel, is located in the throat and is associated with the thyroid and parathyroid glands. This center also governs the nervous system, ears, and voice. The throat chakra is associated with the ability to speak our truth.

The brow chakra, the sixth wheel, is also known as the third eye. This center, located between the eyebrows, is connected with the pituitary gland. The sixth chakra also deals with the eyes, nose, ears, and the hypothalamus, which is part of the brain. The third eye is our sense of awareness, our intuitive self.

The crown chakra, the seventh energy wheel, is found at the top of the head. This center allows direct access to the flow of energy from the universe. The pineal gland is the crown chakra's affiliation with the endocrine system. The crown chakra helps to bring together the connection of body, mind, and soul.

Other Chakras

Two other chakras carry a tremendous amount of importance. The **splenic chakra** is located near the spleen area on the left side of the body just above the waistline. This wheel stores the life force just as the spleen stores blood. Of equal importance is the **etheric chakra** connected to the thymus. This chakra is found on the centerline between the heart and the throat.

Reflexology affects these energy centers in a profound and dynamic sense. Reflexologists work directly with the nervous system as they perform reflexology. They are also dealing with energy and are therefore connecting with the chakras on that level.

PART 2

Getting Started in Reflexology

Nothing is so healing as the human touch.

—BOBBY FISCHER

IN THIS PART, the focus is on getting started in the practice of reflexology. You'll find out how to create a healing environment—from choosing the right space to picking the right chair. You'll explore how to find and use the right props, from the music you play to the foot soak you offer clients. You'll also learn about using essential oils, lotions, powders, and more.

Then, the focus shifts to the mental and emotional. You'll learn about setting your intentions and clearing your energy before you get started. You'll find out how to focus on the task of giving your energy. And you'll get some practical advice on using a calm, even touch and keeping your nails short and your hands clean.

Finally, you'll delve into some basic reflexology techniques, including thumb walking, finger walking, tapping, feathering, and many others. By the time you're done with this part, you'll be ready to move on to giving reflexology a try!

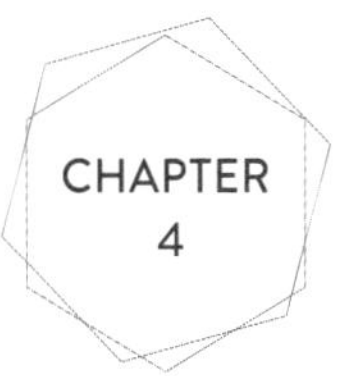

Preparing for Reflexology

"Sacred space" is another way of saying "with intention."
—*S. KELLEY HARRELL*

Reflexology teaches people to reconnect with the feet, to actually honor and pay attention to these wonderful creations. Whether you want to work only on family and friends, or if you would like to practice reflexology professionally, you'll need to create a space conducive to healing. To do so, you must gather the proper items needed to make the most of a session. You don't have to sublet an office or remodel your basement—and you won't have to take out a loan to pay for it! With some care and attention, you can carve out the perfect spot in your own home.

This chapter will show you what you need to create the ultimate relaxation setting for reflexology. You'll learn how to set the mood with music, when and how to use a foot soak, and the various uses of oils and lotions.

Create a Healing Space

So far you've learned how reflexology can relax a person. But where do you perform the reflexology techniques? In the middle of the family room with all the children running around? In the garage among all the tools and bins?

Setting aside an appropriate place to practice this healing art is important. Take a walk through your living area and feel where you begin to relax. Sit in this place and see if it's comfortable to you. Make sure there's enough light—natural, if possible. Check to see if the air is clear; see if there's enough space without clutter. Even if you live in one room, you can be creative with the section where you will be working.

• • • Reflex Points • • •

The rule for space clearing is keeping it simple. Getting rid of clutter is essential. Whether physical, mental, or emotional, releasing old junk allows you to function in balance and harmony. The areas of living and working need to be not only physically clean but also spiritually clean.

Once you have decided where you want to work, use lots of elbow grease and clear out all dust, dirt, and dinginess. Let yourself look through the eyes of the person who will be receiving reflexology in that setting. The size of the area is not important; rather, it's the energy of the space that is key. It should say, "Welcome! Come and relax, put your feet up, and enjoy."

The Right Chair

Reflexology can basically be done anywhere and on anything, but a good chair makes a difference. Here's how to find one that works with your space, goals, and budget.

RV Recliners

Reflexologists use a multipositional recliner, the kind that can be bought in a recreational vehicle (RV) store or website. These chairs are great because they have been created with the thought of saving space as well as providing comfort.

The chairs may cost several hundred dollars, but a higher price does not necessarily equate to a better chair. If possible, sit in the chair before you buy it. Let the chair fully recline while checking to see that the back is down, your feet are up, and your arms are supported. Make sure the frame of the chair is sturdy and know the maximum weight the chair will hold.

The Best Position

Not everyone can rush out to buy a chair; sometimes what is already in the house will work just as well. A recliner or any chair that tilts back will put your receiver in the proper position. The best position is with the head back and legs a bit above chest level. This position supports the back and assists with blood flow. Some people cannot have their head all the way back, so the chair must be adjustable enough to accommodate them.

• • • Reflex Points • • •

If someone is restricted to bed rest, pull a chair up to the bottom of the bed and go to work. If someone is wheelchair-bound, place a stool or hassock in front of the chair and commence with the session. Always check with the person to see if she is comfortable or if she needs a bolster or other implement for support.

A massage or Reiki table will work using pillows or bolsters. The head should be back and resting comfortably, with the legs slightly raised by a pillow placed under the knees and under the calves. The knees must always be supported; never let the knees sag.

If you do not have a reclining chair or a massage table, another solution is to place two chairs facing each other and have the receiver place one foot on your lap at a time. You can use a pillow on your lap for comfort. This is a quick fix and not recommended for every session, but it will do in a pinch.

Proper Props

Pillows and bolsters are necessary tools in reflexology. One of the best pillows or bolsters to acquire is a foam wedge, one that is large enough to slip under the receiver's knees. The wedge has a narrow edge that fits under the knees and a wide edge that supports the feet. The wedge places the feet perfectly in front of the practitioner's chest, so he or she can see the feet and work on them easily. Wedges can be found online and at stores that carry bed and bath products.

Pillows of all shapes, sizes, and thickness are important tools that provide customizable support and assistance in positioning. Some people need pillows behind their head; some need more height or support under their feet and legs. Have a variety of pillows on hand to assist in making the receiver comfortable.

Covers

Blankets are necessary to provide comfort to the receiver. Think about what happens when you really relax: your temperature drops and you feel chilly. This is exactly what happens during a reflexology session. A cuddly fleece or other lightweight throw is often all that is needed. The act of tucking in the receiver as she lies back in your chair is very nurturing, setting the scene for continued trust and acceptance of the work.

Towels can provide additional coverings. After the pillows are positioned, a towel can be placed on top of them. You should arrange the pillows before you lay out the towel, so that all of the surface areas will be smooth and comfortable. Towels can also be wrapped around the feet and may be used under the head for added support.

The Reflexologist's Chair

What about your chair? The exercise ball is a favorite choice, as they come in all sizes and allow complete freedom of movement during the session. Rolling office chairs are great, especially those with seats that move up and down. Drummer stools work too. Some reflexologists prefer chairs with a back, while others like the freedom of backless chairs. Folding camping stools are great. Not only are they the right height; they also travel well. Hassocks are soft to sit on and are also often the right height, allowing you to rest your legs under the chair.

You will know you are at the right height to work if your legs are comfortable and the receiver's feet are at your chest level. You need to be able to move your arms easily without raising your elbows. When beginning a session, check to make sure you are able to see the feet and move your arms freely, and that your leg position feels comfortable.

Music

Music plays a part in working to reduce stress. The key to appropriate sound for reflexology is to find music with soft, even beats and melodious instrumental tones. Music for meditation, massage, yoga, or any healing art is fine.

Peaceful, soothing music used repetitively is best to promote relaxation. If you always play the same music during the reflexology sessions, the receiver will be given a subtle message to begin relaxing every time the music begins.

The use of music is good for the giver too. Recorded rhythm is a subtle reminder to move your body while applying the treatment. Remember, if you move while you are giving, you will protect your body and give a better session.

Foot Soak

Foot soaking is a way to further the caring and guarantee cleanliness. A simple soak with warm water and Epsom salts is a fantastic way to begin a session. The warmth of the water coupled with the soothing relief from the Epsom salts introduces relaxation immediately. A clean dishpan (used only for foot soaking) is a fine implement for the soak. Just use bleach after each soak to sterilize the container.

Starting a session by soaking the feet allows the receiver a few moments to kick back and disengage before the hands-on work begins.

• • • Reflex Points • • •

Sterilizing the equipment used is essential. This simple step to ensure the absolute cleanliness of your paraphernalia promotes the safety of the receivers. Sheets, towels, pans, and hands all need to be properly cleaned and cared for. Strict adherence to these precautions protects the receiver as well as the giver.

Essential Oils, Lotions, and Powders

Reflexology doesn't use much gliding, sliding, or rubbing; therefore, a lubricant is not necessary, though it can be a nice add-on. A pinch of product before the session may help with movement if the receiver's feet are excessively dry or sweaty. If you choose to do this, apply the product to your hands rather than the feet to be worked. You have a wide variety of products to choose from, including essential oils, lotions, and powders. It's important to remember that oils, lotions, and powders should not be combined in a given session. Most reflexologists work with just one consistently and use it at the end of the treatment. Whatever product you choose to use on the feet, if you wish to apply it liberally, do so only after the session is complete.

Essential Oils

The use of essential oils in reflexology has grown in importance over the past few years as practitioners have come to recognize the healing properties of aromatherapy. The many varieties of oils available may be confusing. A rule of thumb is to look for organic oils, those that have been prepared and infused without alcohol. Generally, essential oils are packaged neat (unblended). The practitioner then mixes it with a carrier oil for safe dispersing. The label of an essential oil should read "100 percent pure," which means it is not blended, or "100 percent natural," which indicates there are no synthetic additives. Commercially produced essential oils may contain alcohol. Read all labels before buying any individual or combination oils, and stay away from those that contain additives.

• • • Reflex Points • • •

A guideline for aromatherapy is to understand that less is more. Do not overuse; a drop of pure oil goes a long way. Remember to check with your receiver for any known allergies. If you have any questions about essential oil use, consult a professional aromatherapist.

Lotions

Foot lotions come in all colors and scents and have a thicker texture than essential oils. Specific aromatic oils used for relaxation may be included in the lotions you purchase, either in a blend or singly.

Peppermint and lavender are often the scents used in lotions since they contribute to relaxation. Lotions that contain tea tree oil are good for antifungal and antibacterial use. Generally, lotions are a better choice than oils, as the incidence of reaction is far less with lotions than with pure oils.

Powders

Powders assist in absorption. If your hands or the receiver's feet are sweaty, sprinkle some powder on your hands and go to work! Cornstarch, talc, and alum are all used as a base for powders. The roots from certain underground plants are ground into powder, and the use of these products will not clog pores. The more natural the powder, the better, but good old baby powder works well.

The purpose of the powder is to allow the treatment to move along without interruption—to enable a free transition from one reflex to another. Often powders are scented, which lends an aromatic flavor to the session. Powder applied at the end of a session may be used more liberally than at the beginning of the treatment.

Applying oils, creams, or powders is a way for the giver to connect more deeply with the receiver. Whichever you decide to use, have fun!

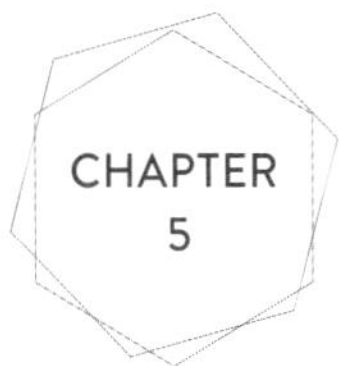

CHAPTER
5

Set Your Intention

Intention is one of the most powerful forces there is. What you mean when you do a thing will always determine the outcome.
—BRENNA YOVANOFF

The right intention allows you to remove all worry from a session. By intending to do the very best and most appropriate work, the experience will be positive. Reflexology cannot hurt anyone, and this fact allows the giver to practice without fear. As a giver, when you perform without fear, you infuse the session with peace and harmony, further empowering the receiver. This chapter is about how to create the right intention not just through your thoughts but with your actions—using a calm touch, keeping your nails short and your hands clean, and focusing on your task. By acting as well as thinking purposefully, you'll create the right environment for healing to occur.

The Importance of a Calm, Even Touch

Touch of any kind should always be even and steady with good pressure and given in a calm, caring manner. Think about what you are doing as you prepare to work on the receiver. A gentle approach allows the receiver to become accustomed to your touch. Remember, you're entering into another person's energy space, so be respectful. As you begin the session, let yourself be calm and honor the receiver, who trusts you. Never push too hard, use tools, or dig in with your thumbs and fingers, even if the receiver asks you to do so.

Clearing Your Energy

Now that you have set your intention, make sure that your energy is clear. Do not bring any of your stress to the session. It is important for givers to practice staying focused in the moment of the giving and not be distracted by any outside interference. While you are in the role of practitioner, remember that you are the good listener, that you are the one who is providing the quiet space and giving permission for the receiver to let go. Practice manifesting a calm and stress-free environment, creating the reality you will demonstrate to your receiver. Ideally, a trusting relationship will develop between the giver and the receiver.

• • • Reflex Points • • •

Meditation and guided visualization are tools that can help you clear out the old junk and create a positive reality. Spend five to ten minutes a day, either early in the morning or last thing at night, becoming still, releasing anxiety and stress. Use meditation and breathing to clear out negativity. Guided visualization is useful in generating the beginnings of this lifestyle.

Focusing On the Task

Once you've set up a workspace, you'll need to prepare an interview format. Reflexology is about touching, and it is imperative to be familiar with the health history of the person you'll be working on. You must also receive permission from the receiver before you begin the session. It is good practice to discuss briefly what is to be expected during and after the treatment. Before you begin working on a new receiver, carefully go over the details of the following list.

1. Create the receiver's history sheet.
2. Ask the receiver to sign a release form.
3. Explain what reflexology is.
4. Explain what will transpire.
5. Discuss the outcome.
6. Give suitable homework.
7. Schedule additional sessions if appropriate.

The receiver's history should include questions regarding current health, allergies, old injuries, and any medications. Find out what the medications are treating, as this will help you to understand what conditions are present. Ask about current stressors and how the person is feeling at the moment. The following list of questions can be a good starting point:

- What causes stress in your life?
- When did you last see your doctor? What for?
- Do you have any current health issues?
- Are you on any medication? If yes, for what?
- Do you visit a chiropractor? How often?
- Do you receive any other adjunct therapies?
- Have you had any past injuries, accidents, surgeries, or ailments?
- Do you have any allergies?
- Do you exercise? How often?
- Are you pregnant?
- What areas of your body hold tension?
- Do you have any discomfort in your feet? If so, describe.
- Have you ever had reflexology before? If so, describe.
- What are your goals in seeking reflexology at this time?

The Release Form

A simple release form indicates that you have been given permission to perform reflexology. A release form should plainly state that you do not practice medicine, you do not prescribe or change medications, and you do not diagnose. Take a look at the following sample release form. It includes the basic information that you should include on your own release form.

LETTERHEAD OF YOUR PRACTICE

To the Clients of Such-and-Such Institute of Reflexology
For your information:

- I am not a doctor or medical practitioner.
- I do not diagnose, treat, or prescribe.
- I am qualified to provide a professional reflexology session for the purpose of stress reduction and the promotion of relaxation. Further, reflexology works with the body to encourage a sustained balance and harmony. Reflexology helps to improve circulation throughout the body.
- I will provide the reflexology session using specific thumb and finger pressure applied to reflex points and areas on the feet, hands, and ears.

You need to know that:

- Reflexology is not a substitute for a medical examination, diagnosis, or any other medical care.
- It is your responsibility to stay current in your medical care and report any changes in your health to your medical practitioner.

I, (insert client's name), understand the above benefits of reflexology. I give my consent to receive reflexology for the purpose of stress reduction and the increase of circulation, as well as the promotion of homeostasis. I understand that this is not a medical treatment, nor a substitute for services as would be provided by my primary healthcare provider. I understand it is my responsibility to provide correct information to the reflexologist with regard to my health. By signing this consent, I give permission to (insert the reflexologist's name) to provide professional reflexology sessions until such time as I wish to discontinue the service.

____

Signature of client/Date

____

Signature of practitioner/Date

Stress and Disease

It's important for a receiver to understand what stress is and what it does. Give the receiver a brief description of stress. Stress is the way people respond to change. The response is registered physically, mentally, emotionally, and spiritually. If a person can adapt to change, then he or she has the ability to flow with the stress. If a person finds change unbearable, then he or she creates resistance. It is this resistance that encourages the growth of congestion and blockage in the body systems.

Point out that stress is essential to life. Explain that stress itself is not what causes the upset to our balance and harmony. Rather, it is the reactions to stress that produce physical upsets. If you react in a negative, combative, hostile, or withdrawn manner, you are allowing the stressors to dig in. This digging in forms an environment that is conducive to the growth of disharmony and disease, be it physical or emotional.

Reflexology is an effective tool for modifying the way people deal with stress. Introducing a positive reaction to stress empowers the recipient. Talk about what to expect during a session, letting the person know that he or she will actually relax and begin to release stress almost immediately.

At the Finish

Once the treatment is finished, it is important to reassess and evaluate what transpired, letting the receiver know what to expect. Ask the receiver how he or she feels at the end of the session and give a reminder to drink water, which will allow the release of toxins to continue. Explain how the session should help the receiver remain relaxed, and encourage a peaceful and uneventful sleep later that evening. Point out that the calming effects should last for a few days. Suggest listening to meditative music for ten minutes a day.

Often, scheduling additional sessions is essential for continuing what has begun in the first introductory session. Encourage the receiver to come back on a regular basis over a period of time, as this routine will provide the receiver with the most benefit.

• • • Reflex Points • • •

Most reflexologists recommend a series of treatments, usually performed weekly over a period of six to eight weeks. At the end of that time, the receiver and the practitioner should reevaluate the receiver's needs. Generally, the receiver then commits to a regular schedule of monthly sessions for maintenance.

Be the Giver

Have you ever been on the receiving end of a service and felt the giver was not really present? Maybe she or he had problems at home, was bored, or was already thinking about what would be happening after you left. Didn't make you feel like returning, right? The point here is that, as a giver, your focus should be on the person who is receiving the treatment and the exercise you are actually performing. The receiver trusts you to be totally engaged. You must be committed to staying focused on the needs of the receiver during the time of the session.

Don't Make a Laundry List

Even though your hands perform the task, your brain needs to be actively present. Your body, mind, and spirit have entered into a contract to provide the best care you can to the person who has entrusted you with his or her feet.

• • • Reflex Points • • •

If you're not present when working on a person, you may miss important cues that the feet offer. You may not recognize tension still held in the body or overlook an area that may need more work. The sense that you are not fully invested in the well-being of the person you are serving will be transmitted.

Information about the receiver is constantly being transmitted through the feet. Your hands pick up the information first. As the session progresses, the texture, temperature, and color of the feet change, alerting you to the physical response. You can see by the facial expression how he or she is feeling during the session.

Give the Gift of Relaxation

Often people begin to unwind by nervously talking. You aren't expected to respond, only to listen. A gentle suggestion to lie back and relax at the beginning could be all that is needed to deter excessive talking. Your job is to deliver a proper treatment with efficiency and compassion. To be effective you need to be available throughout the entire session and constantly aware of the receiver's needs. It is an honor to be the one providing the treatment.

Short Nails and Clean Hands

Reflexologists need to have well-manicured nails and hands. The nails must be short so you can perform your tasks without worry. Nails that are too long may scratch, pinch, or prick the receiver. The best way to prevent transmission of germs is to have clean hands. After trimming the nails, wash your hands with warm water and soap, then rinse with cool water. If you move from feet to hands during a session, wash your hands before the move. Upon completion of the session, wash your hands again.

Using Wax

With all this handwashing, your skin will lose some of its natural oil. Make sure to rehydrate by drinking plenty of water and using a good hand cream. Using a paraffin wax machine on a monthly basis can help restore moisture to your hands and heal cracks in the skin.

Using Wax on the Hands

Wax machines are designed to fit a hand or a foot, singly, into the basin. Clear bars of paraffin wax are melted, creating a hot bath. You dip your hand in completely and then lift it out. The warm wax will form a coating around the entire hand. (Be sure to test the temperature before putting your hand in!)

This process is repeated three to five times, until a firm wax glove is formed. The wax forms a protective coating that encourages the oils of the skin to the surface, helping to mend dry skin and cracks. Keep the wax gloves on for ten minutes. Once you peel the wax off, use a moisturizing cream to reinforce the work of the paraffin. Hands treated in this way feel soft and renewed.

Overuse of the wax can leach moisture from the hands, which can lead to breakdown of the protective outer layer of skin. The recommended time between treatments is approximately three weeks to a month. If you decide to use paraffin treatments, make sure you adhere to the guidelines provided on the packaging.

Using Wax on Feet

A great use of the paraffin treatment is to apply it to the feet you are working on. Do not soak the receiver's feet in the machine, however. Instead, dip a disposable towel or tissue in the hot wax and drape it around the foot that is not being worked on. When you finish with the first foot and are ready to begin on the other, use another disposable towel dipped in the hot wax to cover the foot you have completed. Peel the dry wax off each foot before beginning the reflexology treatment and dispose of it safely.

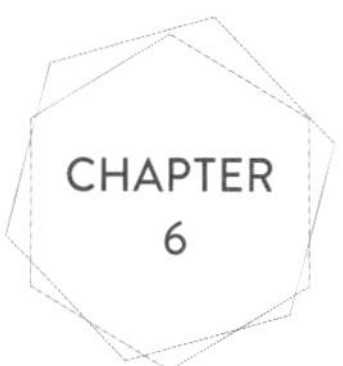

Basic Reflexology Techniques

Our sorrows and wounds are healed only when we touch them with compassion.

—BUDDHA

Reflexology tools are very simple: human hands. Using special techniques with the thumbs and fingers, a practitioner applies pressure in a particular way. Reflexology is fairly straightforward that way, but don't mistake "straightforward" for "easy." You have to practice to learn how to use the techniques correctly and effectively. In this chapter, you'll discover the basic techniques of reflexology, including pressing, tapping, and feathering. In each case, step-by-step instructions are provided to help you visualize how the technique is done. Review the steps carefully before trying the technique. Once you've done so, you can try it on yourself or a willing helper. Don't expect to get it right on the first try—give yourself permission to experiment until you feel comfortable with each technique.

Thumb Walking

Thumb walking is the main movement made during a reflexology treatment. Apply steady, even pressure, moving along slowly over each area. The thumb is a tiny lever and can be used to touch the fine-point reflex areas in the most effective way. Don't concern yourself yet with identifying reflex areas and points. That will come later. You must learn how to walk first.

Learning the Technique

Place one hand, palm down, flat on a table and let your other hand gently rest on it, palm down. Your top hand will be performing the thumb walk; the bottom hand is just the surface on which you'll be practicing the move. Let the thumb of your top hand rest at the top of the bottom hand by the first knuckle joint; let the fingers of your top hand loosely rest above this. Bend your thumb, allowing only the tip of the thumb to touch the skin.

Push off with this thumb so that the pad of your thumb comes in contact with the skin of your bottom hand. After doing this, your thumb will once again lie flat while the rest of the hand lies slightly across the surface, with the fingers relaxed and wrapped easily around the outer edge of the bottom hand. Pull the thumb back up into a bent position, hold down on this spot, and then move forward again. (See Figure 6.1.)

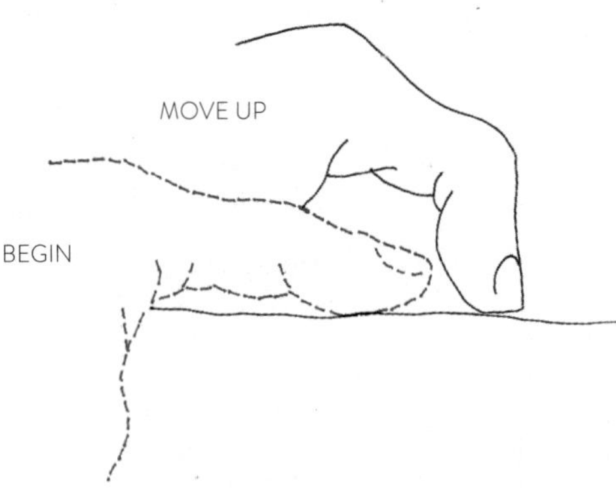

Figure 6.1 Thumb walking is the most important technique you will learn.

The thumb continues to perform this creeping motion with tiny little "bites" across the top of the hand. When you work across the top surface of the hand, the fingers of the top hand will be resting along the top of the bottom hand, above the knuckles.

Each movement is slow and controlled. Pull up at the joint and count: 1, 2, 3. Push down and creep forward on the pad of the thumb and count: 1, 2, 3. Bend up again at the joint, pull back a bit with the thumb, and count: 1, 2, 3. Switch hands and work the same movement across the other hand with the opposite thumb. You do not need to apply extra pressure, just concentrate on the thumb walking right now.

Lift your hands off the table and continue to practice this movement with your hands resting on your lap or on each other. Then turn your hands over and thumb walk along the palm surface, switching back and forth. Allow the fingers of the hand that is working to gently cup the back of the hand being worked while walking the palm with your thumb.

• • • Reflex Points • • •

Three is a very powerful number. Many sacred symbols consist of three shapes, colors, or sizes. The number three has many meanings: harmony, completion through harmony, and the birth of harmony. In reflexology, you will often do each move within a technique three times. With the application of three, you are sure each movement in the process is complete.

Practice, Practice, Practice!

The best way to master this is to practice, practice, and practice some more. Practice on the back of your hand, on the countertop, while you are waiting in line at the supermarket, or while you are sitting at a meeting. Practice on your friends, mom, dad, children, and pets—practice on anyone and any surface available.

Finger Walking

Finger walking is similar to thumb walking; it uses the same motion and form. The index finger—sometimes all the fingers—is bent slightly at the first joint then pushed along in a walking or creeping movement. Practice again on your own hands.

Learning the Technique

Close a hand into a loose fist with the top surface facing up; this is the hand you will work on. Grasp this hand with the other hand, letting your thumb slide between the thumb and index finger of the fisted hand and rest in your palm. The fingers are on top of the hand. While you are using the index finger, the other fingers will rest on top, slightly closed in. These fingers move along without working as the index finger walks down the top of the hand.

• • • Reflex Points • • •

Never use tools to apply pressure. Pushing a pencil or an implement that says it is a "reflexology" tool can hurt the foot! Tools have no feeling; you cannot gauge how deeply they are going into the foot. Remember, fingers and thumbs are all that is needed to do an excellent job. It's not how hard you push; it's where you're working that is important.

Begin at the first knuckle under the index finger of the hand with the closed fist. This is called the hammer position. Begin by placing the finger, tip-surface touching, just below the knuckle. You will be moving away from the fingers down toward the wrist. From the tip touching the hand, the finger is bent with the first joint pushing out. Bend the working finger down at the first joint, pushing forward slightly. This straightens the finger a bit, so that the pad of the finger is touching the surface of your hand. Pull back up into the hammer position. Again the movement is a push-pull motion, creeping along just like the inchworm. This is one finger-walk move.

Walk down the top of the hand, in between the thumb and index finger, in the fleshy section. The thumb will rest under this area; the other fingers are slightly tucked under, just along for the ride. Begin with the finger bent up in the hammer shape, and count 1, 2, 3. Move the finger down into a straight line, with the pad touching the skin pushing forward, and count 1, 2, 3. Pull up into the hammer shape, and pull slightly back again. Imagine you are pinching the skin. You aren't, but it does seem as though you are. Continue this exercise with the finger walking down the fleshy pad and the thumb moving underneath. The thumb holds the underside, providing leverage, keeping the hand steady, and pushing back a bit.

Bring the index finger back to the first knuckle, unfurl your other fingers, and place these fingers at the other knuckles. Bend all the fingers up onto the tips. Move forward ever so slightly, straightening out the fingers as the pads touch the skin. Bring the fingers back up onto the tips; this will pull the skin back toward the knuckles a bit. Move forward again and continue the push-pull movement down to the wrist.

Why the Fingers Are Used

The index finger is used to reach certain reflexes on the top or side of the foot. When the fingers are used, the thumb generally is held in place on the opposite side of the foot to provide leverage. Finger pressure is steady and even, not abrupt or heavy. Using the fingers also gives the thumb a break so the hands don't become tired.

Finger walking allows the area of pressure to broaden. Always move forward with tiny bites. Watch that you are not bending your fingers too much; this will cause your fingers to ache later. Slow movement ensures all the reflexes will be stimulated.

When you use all four fingers at once, you are covering a greater region at one time, which is useful in some areas. The more you practice, the more you will begin to find places on the foot where the index finger or all the fingers are more efficient than the thumb.

Rotation

In rotation, the tip of the thumb is placed directly on the point to be rotated. Using your hands to practice on, turn a palm up and find the space just below the little finger. Whatever palm you choose to work on, let it rest cupped in the other palm. The fingers of the holding hand, which is also the working hand, rest under the knuckles. The thumb is going to work on the palm surface from the little-finger side.

Learning the Technique

Feel under the little finger, on the palm surface. Find the under-surface of the knuckle bone and place your thumb on it. Back up to the edge of the hand and gently thumb walk over the bone, thumb walking along the ball of the hand. You are walking horizontally across the palm. This thumb-walking movement will take about three tiny inchworm bites to reach past this bone. Notice how the tip of the thumb drops into a space after the joint bone is passed over. If you have gone too far, you will find another bony bump, not quite as big as the first.

First, hold the hand steady. Then gently circle in a small rotating motion on this area. Staying right here, continue this move for about the count of three. Now press in and actually rotate the hand a bit, moving it around as the thumb holds the spot. The moving of the hand is minimal; you aren't actually turning the hand for the sake of turning. The movement of the hand is to allow the thumb to move in deeply without much force. To transition from this, move forward in a thumb walk along the rest of the area being worked.

When to Use Rotation

A reflexologist does not always rotate the foot. It depends upon what reflexes or areas are being worked on. Rule of thumb, if anatomically—meaning physically—the foot cannot rotate, such as when working on the toes, do not turn. If the foot can move easily, then go ahead.

Rotation is a technique that allows the thumb to work steadily and directly on a reflex point. The thumb might be walking along when a reflex point is reached that needs more attention. Perhaps the skin is tougher, there is a crunchy feeling under the thumb, or the technique for this particular reflex calls for rotating in on the point. Whatever the reason, rotation feels great to the receiver.

Pressing

This technique uses the entire thumb surface, holding flat along the bottom of the foot on a particular reflex. The thumb is in a holding position, without undue pressure. When pressing is needed, generally after rotating, press down and hold firmly without moving. Pressing allows you to reach an entire reflex surface in a gentle, connected way. This is another technique that, when used properly, will give your thumbs a break.

Pressing on a reflex allows you to feel the subtle shift that will happen as the reflex connects with the energy, releasing any tension in that area. The amount of pressure used with this technique is slight; there is no need to push hard or dig. As the reflex relaxes, the thumb will actually lift up a bit from the skin, an indication to move on.

• • • Reflex Points • • •

Imagine your fingers are your eyes. Once you have learned a basic technique and routine, your thumbs and fingers will be your guide. Through informed touch you will know how much time to spend on a reflex and where to return, if needed.

At times you can rotate the hand as you press, which will broaden the area you are working on. Place your thumb in the center of your other hand. Let the thumb press from the center outward toward the side of the hand. Your thumb is pressing on an imaginary line from the center to the outside edge (lateral side) of the hand. Lift your fingers and turn your hand toward the thumb side of the hand you are pressing on; feel how you stay connected to the reflex, yet allow the area to grow. Try this technique whenever you have a flat area to work, and see when it is effective and when it is not.

Hooking and Pulling Back

This is an advanced move, and it allows you to reach way into a reflex to stimulate deeply without hurting. The hook technique is actually approached in three parts. First, thumb walking is used to move to the reflex, pinpointing the spot. Then rotation is used to zero in on the exact point. Finally, the thumb hooks in on the reflex. Reflexologists pay close attention to the skin under their thumbs to see if the surface is tense or pliable. Only the thumb—on the particular reflexes that you will learn—performs the hooking technique.

Learning the Technique

Hold your left thumb up, curling the other fingers in, giving the thumb plenty of room. The thumb's fleshy pad is facing you. Look at the first section and imagine a line running from the top of the thumb, down the center to the first joint. Find the center of that line and draw an imaginary line across it.

Use your other hand to thumb walk up from the neck of the thumb to the place where the two lines cross. Let the tip of your thumb rest on the crossing point. Now rotation comes into play as you circle in on the exact point. You may feel the point pushing back to you. This is exactly what you want to feel.

• • • Reflex Points • • •

Reflexology is a technical modality that also depends upon the senses of the practitioner. As you become better with the actual technology of application, you will begin to trust what you feel as well. For instance, pushing back is a feeling; you will sense it with time.

Gently continue to circle on the point, using your thumb to apply gentle, steady pressure as the circles move in, targeting the exact spot. Once the rotation has allowed the thumb to touch in deeply, the thumb is then turned halfway around (180 degrees) on the reflex, pushed in, and hooked up.

The hooking movement is done with the tip of the thumb. As the thumb pushes in, it actually hooks on some of the skin. With the hook movement in place, pull the thumb back, as though you have just secured bait on a hook. Don't worry, you cannot hook in too far; the body will stop you.

Hold in this hook-like position, gently pushing in even farther. Please make sure your nails are short, as this technique goes in quite deeply. Hold in this position for a count of three to five, then slowly release as you move on.

The Possibility of Pain

Sometimes the receiver feels a slight flash of pain, which will subside as the point is held. The pain, which feels like a pinprick or the jab of a long fingernail, is an indication that there may be congestion at that particular reflex. If the pain does not abate, move on to the solar plexus reflex (see Chapter 7) where you should press in with your thumb and hold, asking the receiver to breathe slowly and deeply. Release this reflex, return to the painful spot, and hook in again. The pain should be gone or minimal. If the pain continues, just move away from the reflex and continue on with the session.

Holding

There are two types of holding. One holding is what the nonmoving hand does. It is very important to support the foot that is being worked on. The hand holding the foot keeps the foot stable and provides leverage for the working hand. As you switch back and forth during a session, each hand has a turn holding or working.

Hold the foot you are working on by placing the fingers behind the foot with the thumb resting on the sole. If you are working near the top of the foot, hold near the top. If you are working at the bottom of the foot, you will generally hold near the ankle. When you are working on hands, one hand supports and the other works.

Holding the feet in this way provides leverage and support. Leverage allows the thumb or finger doing the work to have a strong hold on the surface being reflexed. The fingers support the foot as the thumb walks on the other side, creating a circle of healing. As the thumb moves, so do the fingers—the leverage and support is always there.

The other type of holding is that of holding on a reflex point during certain techniques. For instance, you may rotate and hold, hook and hold, or press and hold. Remember, reflexology is a steady, smooth system, so holding on a point is integral to this style of work.

When you rotate or press and hold on a point, often the receiver will feel a warm sensation begin to radiate through her body as the thumb stops moving and holds. Holding at the reflex point amplifies the healing effect. With the hook and hold, you are pinpointing a very specific region of the reflex, again creating a direct pathway.

Butterfly

Butterfly is a wonderful two-handed technique used to smooth out an area and to work a bit deeper. It is named the butterfly because the imaginary shape the thumbs make are like the wings of a butterfly. This technique is done with both hands holding on to the foot, with the palms resting on the top surface of the foot and the thumbs on the sole. The movement is with the thumbs; the rest of the hand comes along for the ride. Let the thumbs move in toward the center of the foot and back. Imagine that your thumbs look like butterfly wings as you move in and out.

Learning the Technique

The thumbs move in a less exaggerated thumb walk in toward the center and then quickly slide back to the edge. Move your thumbs up each time you are along the edge, basically making a new line to walk. Your thumbs meet at the center of the sole and then slide back to the edge. The butterfly may be done in a specific area or on the entire foot, depending on where you are in the sequence of the treatment. Remember, unless otherwise indicated, the fingers basically slide along with the hands as the thumbs perform.

• • • Reflex Points • • •

As an effective transition tool, the butterfly technique allows for easy movement as you change from one place to another. At times you may move your fingers as well as your thumbs. In this case, all the fingers and the thumbs are moving in concert from the outside of the foot to the middle.

Practice, Practice, Practice

Hold your hands in the air with your thumbs in finger-walking position. The fingers are slightly bent, tips overlapping, as though resting on the top of a foot. Let the thumbs walk toward each other until they touch. Imagine they are sliding on the foot as you pull them back, move down slightly, and thumb walk in again. Your fingers may have to move away from each other a bit to get the full effect. The important thing is to practice, practice, and practice. Now try this on a foot.

You can butterfly an area or the entire surface of the foot. Start at the top of the foot or the bottom and move both thumbs into the center of the foot with a long thumb-walking stride. The fingers are slightly bent and gently gliding along the top surface. As the thumbs reach the center, gently glide them back to the outside edge of the foot and move up slightly. Continue until the hands reach either the top or bottom of the foot, and either repeat or move on to the next segment.

Karate Chops

Karate chops help with circulation, and they are one of the signals that the session is ending. This technique is done by holding your hands with fingers together and using quick chopping motions in a staccato effect. The sides of the hand contact the bottom of the foot and along the edges as well.

The chopping effect is stimulating, making the receiver feel energized and ready to move. Karate chops are used at the end of the session to help ground the receiver, bringing him or her back to earth. Reflexology allows a person to relax, hovering between dreaming and sleeping. Some receivers do fall asleep! Karate chops bring the receiver back, allowing time and space to reconnect with the present. The tingling sensation often felt as the blood rises to the surface is a lovely way to wake up.

This technique is effective in dealing with heel pain. Quick, sharp, repetitive chops, especially around the heel ridge, stimulate the stressed tissue associated with pain in the heel. Repeated chopping over a length of time helps to strengthen the tendons that have been overused.

Tapping

This is done with the tips of the fingers tapping along the bottom, edge, and top of the foot. Gentle, quick tapping movements assist circulation and again signal closure, either of the session or as a transition on to the next area. Often one hand taps as the other supports the foot.

Tapping is used up the legs and is very effective on the hands as well. Heel pain generally comes from poor walking habits and the long-term use of improper footgear. Tapping along the calf and the sides of the shin stimulates the tissue by increasing blood flow and nerve transmission.

Generally, all the fingers are tapping together. The tapping may be done up and down the foot, usually on the sole, in a rhythmic style. When tapping on the top surface of the foot, most reflexologists tap from side to side, again using all the fingers at once.

Knuckle Press

This is a great move to relax an entire area. With a closed hand, use the length of the fingers in the fist from the second rim of joints to the knuckles. Gently press in as though kneading dough. (See Figure 6.2.) The hand moves over the area in a steady, rhythmic movement. As the press relaxes the area, you can gently rotate the closed fist, getting in even closer and deeper. Always use an even, slow motion with a kneading, circular style. Do not move quickly with this technique; take your time.

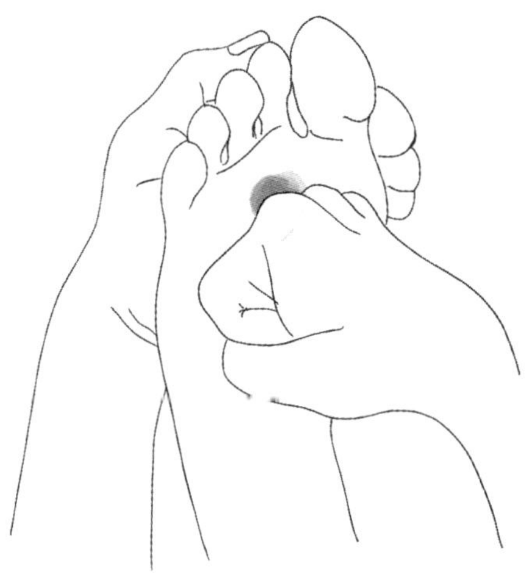

Figure 6.2 The knuckle press is a kneading movement that relaxes large, tough areas.

Let your fisted hands rest down on a tabletop. The fingertips are tucked into the palms, with the second section of your fingers actually resting on the table. Lean your fists up onto the points of the second joints. Now roll from those joints forward, so that the next section of your fingers is now resting on the table. Looking down at your hands you can see the fingertips bending up toward you. Practice rolling back up on the joints and back down on the fingers. This is kneading.

A gentle knuckle press up and down the sole of the foot brings deep relaxation. The press is affecting all the reflexes, allowing for great release. Each time you press into the foot with the knuckles, the message is clear: you are helping the foot relax, and therefore the receiver lets go.

Clapping

Clapping is done with an open hand, actually slapping on the entire foot area. Clap the top surface, the bottom, and the sides as well. The top of the foot is gently clapped, and then this technique is repeated on the bottom of the foot. Both hands can "applaud" the foot at the same time too. At times you may find it is easier to use the palm of the hand, while at other times, the back of the hand is easier.

• • • Reflex Points • • •

The knuckle press is effective in warming up the lung area. Commonly known as the lung press, reflexologists use the flat outside of the fisted fingers and press the entire region. This press is helpful when working on the heel, enabling the giver to relax the entire heel area. Pressing on the heel with the knuckle press relaxes the sciatic line and the lower body as well.

There are two important considerations with this technique, really with every technique. First, always use a steady, even pressure, not a forceful, painful energy. Always work within the comfort zone of your receiver. Traditionally, people have steered away from reflexology because of the misnomer that it has to hurt to be effective. This is not true! Any professional practitioner of reflexology will tell you it's not how hard you push; rather, it is working the reflex areas properly that counts.

Second, see how your hands are feeling as you work on the foot. Does using your palm feel awkward? Try the back of the hand in the area that felt uncomfortable to you. When you clap along the side of the foot, rather than use both hands, let one hand provide support. One hand or both may be used, depending on your comfort with administering this technique.

• • • Reflex Points • • •

The wonderful truth of reflexology is that this is a holistic healing art. Within the definitive guidelines is room for growth and creativity. During the relaxation session you may find you want to do more of a particular style and less of another. Go ahead, experiment and develop your own pattern.

Feathering

This technique is done as a transition and at the finish (after the karate chops, tapping, and clapping). Using both hands with the fingers moving slightly, gently tap off the feet. The fingers do touch the foot, though the touch is light like a feather. On the top of the foot, use the bottom and tips of the fingers. On the sole of the foot, use the backs of your fingers.

Feathering is a stroking, smoothing technique that can be used on the feet or hands. The effect is a soothing, calm feeling. Let your hands stroke the air for a moment, using your hands, and then use your fingers. Then allow the fingers to move in a gentle vibrating manner, as though moving the air about. Again, let your hands smooth the area. Feathering is a combination of both these movements.

Feathering is used throughout the session when you move from one area to another. As the back reflex is finished and you prepare to work the lymph reflex, soft feather strokes allow you to move easily into the section. The feather technique also helps to soothe the area, further promoting the relaxation effect.

PART 3
Foot Fundamentals

Healing is opening what has been closed,
softening what has hardened into obstruction.
—JEANNE ACHTERBERG

IT'S TIME TO explore how to put the basic techniques you learned in Part 2 into action. You'll get instruction on a basic reflexology session so that you can learn how and why to perform techniques such as turning, wringing, and rotating the foot. How to work both feet will also be covered. Then you'll embark on a reflexology journey—using the map of the foot as a map of the body. You'll learn more about therapy zones and meridian lines, which you'll use in your reflexology practice. You'll also discover how to manipulate the toes in order to provide relief from headaches, sinus pressure, and tension in the neck and shoulders. After reading through this part and practicing the techniques, you'll be helping people relax in no time at all!

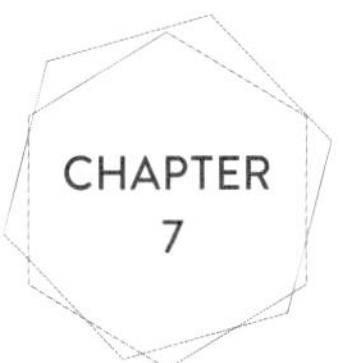

CHAPTER 7

Relaxing the Feet

The human foot is a masterpiece of engineering and a work of art.
—LEONARDO DA VINCI

Caring for your feet is a relatively easy yet essential exercise. To function at their optimal performance level, your feet need to be treated with respect. The greater care you give your feet, the longer they are able to do their job—the job of balance, support, and shock absorption. In this chapter, you'll learn how to start a reflexology session by greeting the feet (preparing them for the session). Then you'll find out how to perform some common—and important!—reflexology techniques, such as turning feet in and out, wringing the foot, and loosening the foot. You'll discover how to use these techniques to relax the spinal reflex and the solar plexus reflex. Finally, the chapter concludes with the specifics of working with both feet.

Greeting the Feet

Before you begin to work on someone's feet, you need to greet the feet. To do this, place both open hands on the bottom of the feet, allowing the hands to rest there gently. You will feel the heat begin to flow between your hands and the receiver's feet. This is a quiet and respectful introduction. Move the hands to the outside of both feet, gently holding until you actually feel the feet relax.

The next step is to place both hands on the right foot, holding top and bottom. Again rest the open hands here, allowing the rhythm of your breath and that of the person in the chair to flow in tune together. The pulse of the foot beats evenly as the heat from your hands penetrates the foot, encouraging further relaxation. Release this foot and let both hands cup the left foot, repeating the same step.

Finally, rest hands on the top of the feet, telling each foot you are ready to begin. Using soft, easy strokes, feather off gently and place both hands on the right foot, sandwiching the foot between the hands. One hand is on top of the foot, and the other is on the bottom, with the open palms resting on the foot. Slightly rock your body back and forth as you also push and pull the foot forward and backward. Everything is done with a count of three to five. This is called dorsiflexion and plantar flexion, relating to the dorsal (top) and plantar (bottom) surfaces of the feet.

The top of the foot is pushed toward the body, and the bottom of the foot is pressed away. The hands rest easily, basically guiding the foot as this motion simulates walking. Many of the relaxation procedures copy motions found in walking. Sometimes receivers will automatically try to help by moving their foot with you. Remind them it is their time to unwind and let go; you will do the work.

Turning Feet In and Out

Stay on the right foot, with both hands grasping the sides of the foot. Slowly turn the foot side to side. Watch the ankle turn in and out—this is the movement you are looking for: an in-out turn with both hands gently guiding the foot. The stationary foot is teased to subtle movement by the guidance of pressure from the holding hand. Here you are again mimicking walking, that side-to-side, in-and-out posture of the foot.

The foot turns in toward the body and then is moved away from the body. The turn is subtle, with the hands positioned to guide the foot in each direction. You will meet with a natural resistance, as the foot can only turn so far in each direction. Let the hands guide the foot as far to one side as is comfortable and then to the other side. The foot will relax and actually feel looser.

Often the person being worked on will try to turn the foot for you. It is easy to feel when this is happening. Reflexologists do not encourage the receiver to help; the receiver is there to relax and release all control. If your receiver is turning her foot along with you, gently suggest that she relax and allow you to do the work. The receiver might not even realize her involvement, so you may have to repeat the reminder a few times.

Wringing the Foot

The next technique is called wringing, which involves wrapping the hands around the foot as though it is a shirt that needs to be wrung out. This simple yet effective relaxation technique relaxes the entire body, as the foot represents the whole body.

Beginning from the bottom, move the hands firmly up the foot, and then move the hands steadily down, wringing all the way. As you hold the foot, your thumbs are on the sole and the fingers are on the top of the foot. The wringing motion is firmly applied—meaning the hands hold the foot closely as they move up toward the toes and down toward the heel. Repeat this three times up and three times down, with your hands remaining on the foot as the wringing is performed. Hold the foot firmly, but do not squeeze or press with great pressure. This is a steady, even move with a healthy grasp of the foot.

Receivers often experience a feeling of warmth spreading through their body at this juncture. You can see a letting go. Some people may close their eyes and begin to drift, releasing tension. Breathing may become more tranquil as the wringing is repeated.

Relaxing the Spinal Reflex

Spinal relaxation is a two-part technique. Hold the right foot with the left hand while using the right thumb and index finger. Starting from the inner edge of the heel, push with the thumb then pull with the index finger along the edge of the inner foot up through the arch to the great toe. Continue with this push-pull movement back down to the inner edge of the heel and all the way up again, doing this three complete times. Use your body to give assistance with a rocking motion; this allows for more effective work.

What you will begin to feel is the actual relaxation of the entire inside edge of the foot, known as the medial edge. The area becomes more palpable, and the color and temperature may change as well. After three or four complete up-and-down moves, the second part of the technique begins.

Place both hands on the inside arch, one next to the other in a grasping style. Both palms are cupping the arch as the fingers wrap around and rest on the top of the foot. Begin to twist each hand in opposite directions while staying directly on the arch line. Move the hands up the inner line as you continue twisting. The top hand moves right, with the bottom hand following. Wring and twist along this edge to the great toe and down to the heel three to four times.

• • • Reflex Points • • •

Moving the body is essential in providing leverage and allowing strength of position to come from the body, not from the hands alone. Effective pressure is best derived from using the entire body. Pushing solely with the thumbs and fingers does not feel as good to the receiver or to the giver.

The receiver will feel warmth spreading up the spine as the twist on the spinal reflex is performed. Give the person you are working on permission to share what is being felt. Throughout the session confirmation is important; the receiver will assist in this process. Watch the receiver for expression in body language as well.

Rotating the Foot

Hold the right foot by cupping the ankle with the left hand and firmly gripping the toes with the right hand. The left hand will provide support, keeping the foot steady as the right hand does the turning. The right hand is folded over the toes so that as you turn the foot, this hand can guide the movement. Using the right hand, rotate three turns clockwise and three turns counterclockwise.

The foot will actually move from the ankle—the turning hand is holding the foot straight and tall as the ankle is gently rotated. The left hand is cupping the back of the heel and ankle. The rotation is slow and defined, and you are assessing as you move the ankle. Check with the receiver to gauge the degree of rotation.

The range of motion in the foot, especially the ankle area, might be limited. The cause of limited range might be an old injury, chronic joint-related issues like arthritis, or some other systemic condition that may affect movement. Do the best you can and be gentle.

• • • Reflex Points • • •

Always keep contact with the foot being worked on. One hand will support and provide leverage while the other performs the working movements. When you stay connected to the feet the receiver feels a deep sense of safety, further allowing for relaxation.

With this movement you begin to actually feel and see the foot, ankle, and even the leg sink down and relax. You have allowed the ankle to be at rest, not having to actively support all the movement.

Loosening the Foot

From the rotation of the foot, move on by tucking the heels of both palms up under the right anklebone. Feel how completely natural this hold is. The hands rest on the sides of the foot as the palms hold close to the ankle. The foot is securely supported, cradled by the palms.

Begin to rock the foot side to side and watch as the foot actually flops around. The more experienced you become with this move, the quicker you can rock the foot. This is a real test of how relaxed the person in the chair is: the more flopping you get, the looser the receiver is.

Move your hands down now to the heel, still in the same cupping fashion. This time the palms hold the heel as you rock the foot. The side-to-side movement will not be as pronounced; the foot does not move as much from this angle. Still, you can see how the foot and ankle have let go of the control and completely surrender.

Stretching

While your hands are resting at the heel, let the right hand reach under and cup the entire heel. The left hand holds across the top of the foot just at the ankle, securing the foot in a safe grip. Keeping the leg straight and resting down on the pillows, picture the hip connected at the end of the leg you are holding. Using very steady, even, and light pressure, pull straight toward you to the count of three. Stop and hold for a count of three to five, then release.

This is mobilizing the hip, which in turn is stretching the back. The hip is often a tight, immobile area of the body. Passive stretching is used to release tight areas. For instance, this stretch helps relieve congestion in the joint. People love this technique, as it is relaxing to the entire body.

• • • Reflex Points • • •

Be very careful when stretching. Do not overpull, and remember to keep a straight line, with no up or sideways movement in the pulling. The object is to mobilize the hip joint, not the knee. Check with the receiver to make sure there is no discomfort in the knee or elsewhere.

Stretching is connected to breathing. Every good stretch generally includes a deep inhaling breath, followed by a long releasing breath. We breathe in as we stretch and exhale as we return from the stretch. Are you getting the picture here? This technique, and all the techniques that you are learning from this book, deal with relaxing, releasing, and letting go.

Greeting the Solar Plexus Reflex

The solar plexus reflex is one of the most powerful reflexes. Whenever a reflex is painful, anywhere on the foot, working the solar plexus reflex may lessen or even remove the pain. It is situated under the ball of the foot, exactly in the center of the foot. You will notice that the thumb fits perfectly into the indented space found there.

This technique is used in the warm-up, during the session, and in the cooldown phase as well. Become familiar with this technique and the reflex. During a session, the solar plexus reflex is an area you press as you transition from one section to another.

Hold the right foot with your left hand, bending the foot from the top to create a hollow space under the ball of the foot. Place the right thumb into this space, pressing in firmly and at the same time pulling the foot down over your thumb. Ask the receiver to take a slow, deep breath in and then exhale slowly, imagining the breath coming out through the feet. The solar plexus press is used to release pent-up tension. This technique is also used as a transition from one segment to another.

Once the breath is released, let the receiver relax and breathe normally. While he or she is breathing deeply, your thumb is held firmly in place. As normal breathing resumes, slowly remove the thumb. Then repeat these steps on the left foot.

Working Both Feet

There are two occasions where reflexologists work back and forth between the feet. The first is during the relaxation sequence and the second is during the cooldown. Generally, they work the entire right foot and then the entire left foot. Relaxing both feet before beginning the session allows the body, mind, and spirit to become totally involved. In this way, you are giving the message to the receiver that it is time to let go of the control and relax.

Once the feet are both relaxed, return your attention to the right foot. Most of the body's processes work from right to left; therefore, you will follow the way the body works. Energetically, the right side is the past and the left is the present. Working from right to left allows the receiver to let go of the past to heal the present.

• • • Reflex Points • • •

Once the treatment portion is complete and the cooldown phase begins, it is fine to move back and forth from one foot to the other. Have fun and remember there is no wrong way, only better ways.

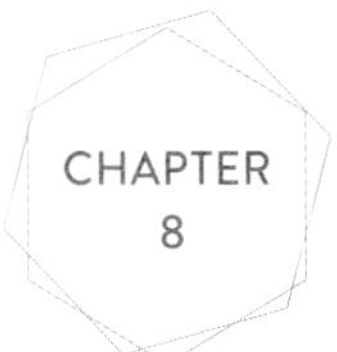

The Foot Is Connected to the Body

Think of the magic of that foot, comparatively small, upon which your whole weight rests. It's a miracle.
—MARTHA GRAHAM

Reflexology is a wonderful treatment modality. When it is applied correctly you cannot hurt anyone; you can only help. It is a privilege to help others relax and access their own healing ability. Through the steps and guidelines supplied here, you will learn the basics and perhaps even become interested in further study. In this chapter, you'll refresh your memory regarding the reflexology zones of the feet as well as the meridian lines. You'll be encouraged to view the foot as the map of the body in order to visualize the correspondences between points on the feet and points in the body. Then, you'll learn how to perform a reflexology session using the whole foot in a logical sequence, applying specific techniques along the meridian lines of the foot.

Remembering the Imaginary Guidelines

As described in Chapter 3, zones and meridians run through the feet. One group is the ten longitudinal zones. Five zones run on each side of the centerline of the body. Each foot is divided into five zones that run through the entire body from head to toe. The great toe represents the major reflexes of the head, so that toe is also divided into five zones.

Zone one begins in the great toe and runs up the body to the brain and then down the arm to the thumb. Zones two through five run the same way, from the corresponding toe to the corresponding finger (for example, zone two runs from the second toe through the body to the head and out to the index finger).

The right side of the body is reflected only on the right foot, and the left side of the body is on the left foot. In the theory of zone therapy, no crossing over to the opposite side of the body occurs.

The Meridians

The twelve meridians are another set of guidelines, with six beginning or ending in the feet and six beginning or ending in the hands. The meridians are curved lines running through the body covering different areas. They, too, are represented on both sides of the body; however, since the lines zigzag back and forth, the reflexes are found on the lines, not in any zones.

The Horizontal Lines

Another set of imaginary guidelines indigenous to reflexology is the transverse lines that divide the sole of the foot into four distinct sections: the shoulder line, the diaphragm line, the waistline, and the sciatic line. (See Figure 8.1.)

• • • Reflex Points • • •

The tendon that runs from the diaphragm line to the heel line is another guideline. This line is used to divide the foot in two. As you work, you will often designate areas to either side of this tendon.

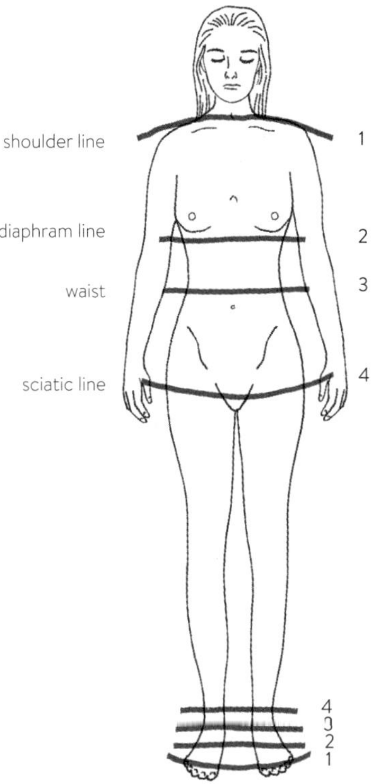

Figure 8.1 The imaginary horizontal lines separate the body into sequential working sections.

Picture the Foot As a Map of the Body

When you look at the feet that are facing you, it is easy to imagine the shape of a body superimposed over those feet. The natural shape of feet resembles the curves and lines of the body. The mirror image found on the feet maps the placement of organs, glands, bones, and muscles.

Reflexology Charts

Reflexologists have a favorite foot chart or map that they use. Often, the chart is the one they trained with, perhaps with additions of their own. The reflexology chart, along with the reflexology technique, has evolved. The more that is learned about the body, energy, and other areas of traditional practice, the more reflexology will continue to adapt and change. (See the charts in Appendix A for examples.)

Corresponding Body Parts

The feet are a map of the body, and every reflex corresponds with an organ or body part.

- The toes are all the head reflexes and all the elements involved with the head, including the sensory organs, brain, endocrine glands, and sinuses. Whatever is on your head is found on the toes.
- The base of the toes equals the neck reflex, including the glands and lymph. The shoulder reflex is found under the toe necks and wraps around from the sole to the top of the foot.
- The ball of the foot, the area that is nicely padded, houses the chest reflexes with all the related organs: heart, lungs, bronchioles, and breast.
- The corresponding area on the top of the foot represents the upper back. There are more lymph reflexes in this area as well.
- From the ball of the foot to about the center of the heel is where all the reflexes to the internal organs and glands that relate to the center of the body are found.
- The remaining top of the foot relates to the lower back.
- The arch line of both feet holds the spinal reflex. The reproductive and pelvic regions are represented along the inside and outside of the foot, from the heel up to the ankle.
- The hip, knee, and leg reflexes as well as the sciatic nerve reflex are found along the underside of the ankle to the outside of the anklebone.
- More lymphatic regions are found running up the center back of the leg.
- Along the outer edge of the feet is the area that represents the musculoskeletal system.

• • • Reflex Points • • •

All the guidelines on the foot help you to locate reflex points. These guidelines and referral areas remind you of the structure of the body while you are working on the feet. Reflexologists learn these aids early on, and they become a natural piece of their work.

A Logical Sequence

Reflexology is a whole body concept. This means that when you work on a person's feet, you work all of the reflex points, not just the area representing a problem. You will begin at the top and move down the entire body, as each point is found on the feet.

Once you have created a healing space, set your intention, and relaxed the feet, you are ready to begin. You will first work completely through the entire sequence on the right foot, and then work through the sequence on the left foot. Save the cooldown section of both feet until the end.

Begin with the toes since they represent the head and neck. Working with the head reflex as the beginning focus allows you to continuously recognize the mirror image of the body as it is represented on the feet. Memorizing the foot map becomes easier if there is a logical sequence to perform. Even though the feet carry around the body, the operating signals come all the way from the head.

As you work your way down, you'll next come to the base of the toes, which are secondary support reflexes. Then move into the ball of the foot, which also includes the long bones of the foot. As you work the sole area, you'll also work the top of the foot. From here you'll go to the arch, covering the upper and lower sections and the top and bottom of the foot. The heel area is next, and then you finally move to the inner and outer sides and ankle areas.

The Shoulder Line

The shoulder line is the demarcation of everything in the body from the shoulders and above. The toes are the face, with the great toe reflecting the major reflexes and the other toes offering support with secondary reflexes. The great toe has reflexes for the pineal and pituitary gland, as well as points for the nose, eyes, ears, brain, forehead, and inner ear. All the toes have reflexes for sinus, teeth, lymph, hair, and the back of the head. The toe necks are equally as important, as they represent the neck area and the glands found there. Of course, the shoulder is also represented.

The great toe is also divided into five zones, denoting all the zones found on the foot and in the body. Remember, in zone therapy the ten zones run through the body, meeting in the head, hands, and feet. The head holds all ten zones, while the feet and hands each have five.

• • • Reflex Points • • •

The great toe, also known as the big toe, holds many reflexes. Just as important is the fact that this toe is part of the medial column, a group of sixteen bones that are key to maintaining our balance and providing shock absorption.

There are many key meridian points above the shoulder line as well. The liver meridian starts at the base of the great toe. The gallbladder meridian passes through the body, ending at the fourth toe. The bladder meridian ends at the little toe. The spleen meridian starts at the center of the great toe. Lastly, the stomach meridian ends at the top of the second toe, with branches to the great toe and third toe.

The Diaphragm Line

The diaphragm line runs along the end of the ball of the foot. This line is representative of the diaphragm muscle that runs across the chest. The areas of the body that are between the shoulders and the diaphragm have symbolic reflexes on the foot. These reflexes are both on the top of the foot and on the bottom.

The organs and other parts of the body linked to this area are sinus, teeth, secondary nose and thyroid reflexes, some of the bronchi, lungs, solar plexus, a section of the thoracic back, and the areas of lymph.

The Waistline

The waistline guideline is found in the center of the arch. The shape of the foot actually helps to locate this line. Look at the outside of your foot. Follow the little toe down the side until you come to a bump. This bump is about halfway down the outer edge; it is the bottom edge of the long bone known as the fifth metatarsal.

The parts of the body represented here are everything from the diaphragm to the waist. This refers not only to the front of the body but to the back part as well. The reflexes for the stomach, pancreas, pyloric sphincter, duodenum, liver, gallbladder, spleen, middle back, adrenals, and top of the kidneys are in this center area.

All the zones run through here as well as the meridians, which connect this section with all the other sections of the foot and thus the whole body. The difference with this area is the location of reflexes. Not all reflexes are found on both feet; here some are on the right foot and some are on the left foot. For instance, the liver, gallbladder, duodenum, and pyloric sphincter reflexes are on the right foot. The spleen reflex is found only on the left foot.

Sciatic, or Heel, Line

This line is easily found, as it is located at the top of the heel. Look at the bottom of your foot. Do you notice how the beginning of the heel seems to have a slightly different color? This line becomes the imaginary guideline. In this area are found all the reflexes from the waist to the tailbone.

The Organs Reflected

All the organs below the waist are found reflected in this section of the foot. However, this area has reflexes for certain parts on one foot and different parts on the other foot. For instance, the right foot reflects the right side of the small and large intestine, and the left foot represents the left side of these organs.

This guideline is itself a reflex. When you thumb walk across the heel line you are affecting the sciatic nerve. The sciatic nerve is the largest nerve in the body; it travels from the sacrum and down the back of the leg to the knee. There, it divides into smaller branches as it runs down the lower leg and into the foot.

• • • Reflex Points • • •

Stimulating a reflex point in any zone in this area will of course stimulate the entire zone. The spleen, bladder, kidney, stomach, gallbladder, and liver meridians pass directly through this area.

Heel to Heel

The heel, or sciatic, line brings us to the end of the reflexes found in the abdominopelvic cavity. However, the section between this line and the end of the heel is important. This part of the foot reflects the lower back, legs, feet, and hips. Unfortunately, this secondary access to the lower extremities is an area often forgotten in foot care.

Many people suffer from dry heels with cracked and broken skin, swelling, and/or bone spurs in this section. In a reflexology session, this area of the foot is included, often using this space as a transitional spot. Reflexologists generally use the knuckle press here, as this can be a tough section to work.

The Tendon Line

The tendon that runs from the heel to between the first and second toes is used as a guideline. This line helps to divide the foot, offering a landmark to work in toward as you thumb walk across the sole of the foot. This tendon is one of many found in the sole of the foot, but it is not difficult to locate.

Feel along the sole of the foot, letting your fingers trace a line from the ball down to the heel line. Feel the tautness along this particular tendon; there is actually a line you can feel vertically down the sole surface. Have the receiver flex her toes; you will notice that the tendon line actually presents itself to you.

• • • Reflex Points • • •

Direct pressure on this tendon line will cause pain and undue stress to the tissue. Always use even, gentle pressure when performing reflexology. The use of undue pressure at any time not only causes unnecessary pain but also could overstimulate an area.

Feel the area as the toe is flexed. This visual appraisal is important. If during a session you notice the tendon is visible, instruct the recipient to relax. Often people want to help or become too involved, tensing the muscles in their body. Help the receiver to relax by performing gentle knuckle pressing or by turning and wringing the foot.

Take note that you do not apply pressure directly on this tendon. The tendon is a guideline, directing you in your approach. There are reflexes that fall on one side or the other with regard to this line. This tendon line helps you to find exact points and to remember where you are on the foot in relation to the body.

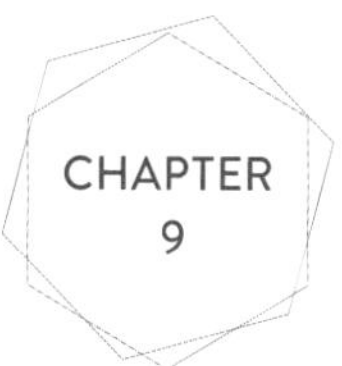

CHAPTER
9

Foot and Body Correspondences

The number one root of all illness, as we know, is stress.
—*MARIANNE WILLIAMSON*

Many theories inform reflexology. As wide and varied as some of these theories may be, there are constants as well. The divisions of the feet and representation of reflex points are generally similar. Many reflexologists today recognize the physical and energetic connection of the work, and understand that footwork encompasses a vast amount of ever-changing information. In this chapter, you'll learn how the foot mirrors the body, how working the left foot affects the left side of the body—and how working the right foot affects the right side of the body. Then you'll delve into the details of the foot's structure so that you can learn to use the bones of the foot as guidelines when you practice reflexology.

Right Foot, Right Side; Left Foot, Left Side

From our head to our toes, the left and right side are basically the same, except for a few differences. The right side contains the liver, gallbladder, pyloric sphincter, duodenum, jejunum, and ileum. This side also contains the ileocecal valve, cecum, appendix, and ascending colon, as well as the right hepatic flexure. These organs are essential in the process of digestion and elimination.

The left side of the body duplicates the right in most areas. The differences occur in the left region of the upper abdomen, which houses the spleen, and in the intestinal area. The unique areas of the left side of the body are the descending colon, the sigmoid colon, and the reflex for the rectum.

It's That Mirror Again

The mirror image of the body is reflected on the feet. A picture of the body superimposed over the feet lends credence to this image. The head sits at the toes, and the rest of the body basically follows along, with the center of the body reflected on the inner sides of each foot. The outer edges of the feet represent the outside of the body.

The Mirror Is Energetic

Of course the mirror is not only physical but energetic as well. There are many theories connecting the body with the feet. Some have already been discussed in the preceding chapters, such as zone therapy and meridians.

Repetitive Treatments

Repetitive treatments seem to store a memory within the sensory system that quickly comes to the surface during a session. The first time a receiver is given a reflexology treatment he or she probably has no idea what to expect. The receiver may have only the understanding that reflexology involves relaxation techniques. Regardless, the person in the chair often cannot keep her eyes open much past the relaxation part of the session. Throughout the treatment the receiver may talk, sleep, remark how relaxed she or he feels, or provide any variety of such responses. By the time the session has ended, the receiver is likely ready to schedule a return appointment.

As you practice you will find that the people you work on will become enamored with reflexology, always eager for you to work on their feet. Remember, the more you practice, the better you become. Some people find relief of chronic pain through continued reflexology treatments. Although you do not treat any condition with reflexology, continued release from stress can help manage pain.

Repeat sessions seem to create a pattern within the body that recognizes reflexology as a tension reliever. The mirror here is one that reflects the memory of relaxation due to stress release. The entire body relaxes during a session, even the conscious mind. Generally, the receiver slips into a semi-dream state, aware yet relaxed. Many people who repeatedly receive reflexology report that they continue to feel relaxed between sessions. It seems that the effects of this modality allow for long-term, sustained relief.

Expect the Unexpected

Let's say you've begun to practice on others. You understand the concept of zone therapy. Therefore, you realize that what is on the right side of the body reflects on the right foot and vice versa. You have relaxed both feet, and you are working on the right foot. As you reflex the shoulder point on the right foot, the receiver relates that he is experiencing a feeling in his left shoulder.

How can this be? Remember, always listen to the receiver; it is his or her body! "But, but," you think, "this is impossible." No, it is not impossible. The person in your chair is affected by the work from the right foot not only on the right side of the body but at times on the left side as well. Are you confused?

The Integration of Somatic Therapies

Reflexology is not only zone therapy; it is also an integration of many somatic therapies. The concept of meridians is definitely involved. Meridians are reflected on both sides of the body just as zones are; yet the areas are not restricted to a given side. As you work on one side of the body in an area where a meridian runs through, the energy may connect to the opposite side of the body. For example, any of the meridians out of the feet will at some point run near the shoulder, and all of the meridians of the hands run through the shoulder.

Another area where you may see opposite areas affected will be the reflex connections with the head. The right side of the brain affects the left side of the body, and the left side of the brain affects the right side of the body, and this may be reflected in the session as well.

Basic Guidelines

Whatever the reason for an unexpected response, these basic guidelines will help you to provide an appropriate treatment:

- Trust in yourself.
- Believe the receiver.
- Listen openly and intuitively.
- Know you are helpful.
- Go with the flow.
- Have respect for the work.
- Be patient and keep learning.

The body is an incredible creation, alive with feeling, physically as well as emotionally. All areas of the body have sensory receptors, allowing the skin to feel the slightest touch to the heaviest pressure. The skeletal muscles also receive sensory input, which allows us to have feeling inside the body as well. All of the body is connected, not just the direct spot you may be touching.

Explanation of Bones As Guidelines

The bones of the feet give reflexologists clear guidelines to perform their trade. Reflexologists also work on the lower leg because the tendons, ligaments, and muscles that connect into the foot are key to movement. The foot contains twenty-eight bones, four layers of muscles, twelve tendons, and over one hundred ligaments. There is distinct anatomical terminology for the bones of the foot, and there are specific terms used to explain direction and movement. The bones of the foot are separated into three regions. These regions are the proximal tarsus, the intermediate metatarsus, and the distal phalanges.

The Proximal Tarsus

The tarsus consists of seven tarsal bones that form the back and ankle region of the foot and the lower arch.

1. Talus, the anklebone
2. Calcaneus, the heel bone
3. Cuboid, a cube-shaped bone
4. Navicular, a bean-shaped bone
5. Medial cuneiform, the inside bone
6. Middle cuneiform, the middle bone
7. Lateral cuneiform, the outside bone

The anklebone, or talus, is actually situated between the two bones of the lower leg; this bone is the first weight-bearing bone to receive pressure during the action of walking. The heel bone, or calcaneus, is the largest and strongest of the foot bones. The heel takes half of the weight from the ankle, and the other tarsal bones carry the remainder of the weight during walking.

These bones are the guidelines for the lower-body reflexes. The heel represents the lower back, especially the sciatic reflex. Part of the intestine reflexes are also housed in the heel. The talus has access reflexes for the fallopian tubes and the vas deferens, and reflexes for the lymphatics.

The navicular bone sits on top of the foot and is sandwiched between the talus and the three cuneiform bones. The reflex for the lower back does reach this bone, as do the reflexes for the lymphatics. The cuneiforms come along the top of the foot from the inside edge, representing the lower back.

The Intermediate Metatarsus

The metatarsus is made up of five metatarsal bones. These bones are known as I through V, with number I being the metatarsal bone near the inside edge. These bones have three parts: a base, which touches the tarsal bones; a shaft, which consists of the length of the bone; and the head, which touches the bottom of the toe digits. The reflexes involved with the metatarsal bones are all those found from the diaphragm line to the sciatic line, whether these points are on the top or bottom of the foot.

The Distal Phalanges

There are five phalanges of the foot, also known as I through V. Four of these toe bones, numbers II through V, have three parts: the base, which touches the metatarsals; the middle; and the head, which is the tip of the toes. The great toe, also known as the hallux or big toe, has two phalanges. The bones of the great toe are heavier and bigger than the other toe digits. The great toe contains a base and a head. The reflexes dealing with this section of the foot are those found from the shoulder line up to the tips of the toes.

• • • Reflex Points • • •

Two small bones, the sesamoid bones, are connected to the first metatarsal head. These bones are actually in the tendons and sit on the underside of the metatarsal. Sesamoid bones seem to appear in areas that take a great amount of pressure. Some people have sesamoid bones in their little toe as well.

Arches of the Foot

There are three arches of the foot, formed by the bones. The arches give the foot the ability to support and balance the body. Leverage for walking comes from these arches as well. Although these structures are called arches, these formations are not immovable. The action of walking produces an application of weight and then a lifting off of this weight. The arches act like a spring, providing shock absorption.

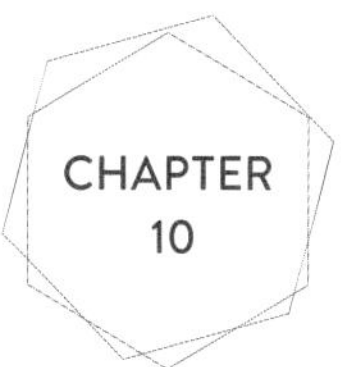

CHAPTER 10

The Toes Know

Cure sometimes, treat often, comfort always.
—*HIPPOCRATES*

As you are now aware, every reflex in your foot is connected to every part of the body. As you perform reflexology you will assist the body in maintaining a well-balanced level of living. Any situation—physical, emotional, or intellectual—can effect a response that may manifest into a physical reality. Reflexology helps the receiver release those responses. In this chapter, the focus is on the toes, the part of the foot that corresponds with the brain. You'll look at how to perform various techniques that can help offer a receiver relief from headaches, sinus congestions, and tension in the neck and shoulders.

Thumb Walking the Toes

Start by holding the right foot with your left hand while the right hand does the walking. The left hand will support the foot. Begin with the great toe and slowly take small bites as you thumb walk along the edge of the toe up to the top. Walk across the top of the toe and down the other edge into the toe web. Use your left hand to separate the toes, as the thumb walking down into the web will feel awkward at first. Your right thumb can only go down so far along this first inside edge. When you feel that the thumb cannot go any farther, turn and thumb walk up the ridge of the next toe.

Thumb walk up each toe, walk across the top, and walk down the other side to each web. Once you reach the outside of the little toe with your right thumb, switch hands. Now the right hand becomes the holding hand, and the left hand does the work. Thumb walk back along the ridges and down into the web of each toe until you again reach the great toe.

• • • Reflex Points • • •

When your thumb makes the turn, it will feel as though you are swiping in between the two toes. Be patient. At first you will feel like you are all thumbs, but this will pass. View this process as walking up the mountain, across the plateau, and down the mountain into the valley. From the valley, it is back up the mountain again.

Walking the Zones on the Great Toe

After you have walked to the farthest side of the great toe, switch hands so that you are working with your right thumb. Use your left hand to support the right foot by holding the top half with your palm and gently wrapping your fingers and thumb around the foot. Now you should imagine the great toe divided into five zones; you will be walking each zone on the great toe.

Start at the base of the great toe and thumb walk up on the flat sole surface of the toe. This is zone one. Bring your thumb back to the toe neck and thumb walk up in an imaginary line right next to the first walk up. This is zone two. Keep bringing your thumb back to the toe neck and walk up each zone; this will include the side of the toe as well. Do not drag your thumb back to the neck, just take it back smoothly and walk up the next zone. After the last zone, use your thumb to rotate on top of the toe, moving in small circles, as you stimulate the brain reflex.

The Remaining Toes

From the great toe, bring your right thumb to the base of the second toe, the plantar (bottom) side, and thumb walk up to the tip of the toe. Bring the thumb back to the toe neck and walk up to the top again. Rotate and hold on the top of the toe. Remember, rotation is using your thumb in a small, circular motion on one area. As you are holding, feel through your thumb how the surface of the toe begins to give, responding to the treatment.

The remaining four toes each have about two lines for you to walk up. These are not zones; rather, they are imaginary lines you are picturing to guide you through the toes. At the top of each toe, circle and hold, then move on to the next toe. Repeat until all toes have been thumb walked in this manner. As you complete the baby toe, switch hands and walk back along each toe, repeating the movements with the left thumb. The right hand becomes the holding hand, giving support and leverage.

Walking the Tops of the Toes

Don't forget the top (dorsal) surface of the foot! The reflexes on the top side reflect the back of the head. Holding the right foot with your left hand, let the right thumb rest along the bottom side of the toes. This thumb will provide leverage while the tops of the toes are being worked. Using your index finger, walk down the top of the toe to the base. Bring your finger back to the top and walk down again. Repeat once more; then move on to the next toe. Complete this movement on all the toes and then switch and walk back.

• • • Reflex Points • • •

What is the toe neck? The toes are shaped a bit like our head, with the larger portion of the toe relating to the part of the skull that houses the brain. The head of the toe is bigger than the lower region of the toe, which is why we refer to this lower region as the toe neck.

Working the Necks of the Toes

After walking all the toes along the ridges, the plantar surface, and the dorsal surface, you will now move into the area that represents the neck. With the left hand holding the right foot, use your right thumb to walk the neck of the great toe on the bottom of the foot. Move in very little sections from the outer edge of the toe in toward the next toe. Bring your thumb back and repeat with tiny bites along the neck for several swipes across. The toe neck will probably feel stiff under your thumb, so try walking until this area feels less tight.

Allow your thumb to rest as you walk with your index finger along the neck surface of the toe on the top of the foot. Again, take tiny bites as the finger walks to the edge of the toe, and then bring your finger back to repeat again.

Finally, with both thumb and index finger, walk together toward the other side of the toe. The thumb is on one side of the toe, and the index finger is on the other side. Let the index finger rest at the base on the top of the foot as the thumb actually walks in between the first and second toe, at the base. Once completed, you will have worked the entire neck reflex.

Thumb Walking the Toe Joint

Each toe tapers into its neck, which connects to a joint at the base of the toe. This second joint of the toe is called the metatarsophalangeal joint. You can also refer to this area as the MTP joint. The MTP joint is that which bends the toes at their base. There are many reflexes in this region.

Hold the right foot with your right hand; you will be using your left thumb for this area. Thumb walk across this joint from the baby toe to the end of the second toe. Bring the thumb back and walk along this joint again. You are walking right in the folded area, where the necks of the toes bend. Switch hands. With the left hand holding the foot, use your right thumb to walk in the joint from the great toe out to the little toe. Repeat this thumb-walking process a few times.

Again with the left thumb, walk into each web starting with the web between the fifth and fourth toe. As the thumb moves into the web, you will feel a hard ridge. Stop here, rotate, and hold gently; do not push. Rotate and hold into each web, ending in the final web next to the great toe.

From the baby toe, thumb walk through again in the ridge with tiny, slow bites, using your left thumb. Then let your thumb begin to move along under the ridge into the fatty part of the foot. This area is directly under the joint, and you will walk here from the little toe to the great toe. Bring your thumb back under the little toe and stay along this region as you walk back to the great toe again. Switch hands and walk back and forth a few times.

Using your right hand as the holding hand, rest your left hand along the outer edge of the foot, with the fingers along the top part of the foot. With your left thumb, walk the space along the outside edge of the foot between the shoulder line and diaphragm line. Then, with your first two fingers, walk on the top surface of the foot from under the little toe to under the third toe. Bring the fingers back to the edge and repeat.

Hooking Specific Reflexes at the Top of the Foot

The reflected image of the shoulder is on the bottom surface of the foot as well as the top and side. There are two areas at the top region of the foot that you will hook. To refresh your memory on the hooking technique, remember to walk in and hold on the spot. Begin to rotate slowly, staying on the reflex point. As you rotate with gentle, steady circles, let your thumb feel the spot underneath. The area should begin to welcome you. Once you feel you have moved in to a comfortable level, push and turn using your thumb as a hook.

Place your left thumb along the outside region, exactly where you walked along the edge, between the diaphragm and shoulder line. Push in easily on the side of the foot where your thumb is. The area under the little toe on the bottom of the foot will actually form a small curvy line next to the bone you feel in that spot. Walk across this area gently, and hook into the space the line has made. Your thumb fits cozily into this spot. Hook and hold.

The great toe has a reflex you hook into as well. Look at the great toe and focus on the first joint. This part of the toe seems big and shaped rather like a head. Imagine a line drawn from the center tip of the toe down to the crease where the neck begins. Now picture another line crossing this vertical line a smidgen above the center of this section of the toe.

Place your right thumb on the spot where the two lines cross. Gently begin to rotate on this spot. Sometimes you may actually feel what seems like a small pea shape at this center cross point. When you feel ready, push in at this spot, hold, and turn so you can hook up with your thumb.

• • • Reflex Points • • •

You might feel a small pulse as you work this area, especially while you are holding on the reflex. Don't worry! This is great; it is the reflex talking back to you! It's a confirmation of a job well done, letting you know you are on the right spot.

Relief from Headaches

Sometimes a person may come to a session with a headache. Whatever the reason, reflexology does help us deal with such pain. A tension headache may result from an upset at work or worry over bills. For some, this type of headache comes after a crisis; the headache is part of the release. Often a headache is a learned response. Whatever the background cause of the tension, reflexology works to bring about balance.

Negative response to tension upsets the natural flow of energy, disrupting homeostasis. A reflexology session helps to restore the vital energy necessary for harmony. The reflexes of the toes contribute to letting go of tension and the return to whole health.

The toes represent the head. The great toes are the entire head, with all the endocrine glands, eyes, ears, nose, throat, brain, teeth, sinuses, and all the anatomical parts of the head. The other toes support the great toe. Some have secondary reflexes, and all have sinus reflexes as well as lymph, teeth, hair, brain, and neck reflexes.

Whatever the cause, reflexology is an appropriate adjunct in support of pain relief. As you help people relax, they become less fearful and less tense, better able to deal with the origin of their pain.

The Toes and Sinuses

The toes are also representative of the sinuses. As you thumb walk along the ridges and up the flat surface of the toes, you are stimulating the sinus reflexes. Thumb walking on the sides of the toes allows you to affect the sinuses in the cheekbones. Thumb walking on the bottom of the toes affects the sinuses found above the eyebrows, on either side of the nose, and those behind the nose.

There are eight nasal sinuses in the head. These little air-filled cavities help to balance the skull. The neck is small in size compared to our heavy heads. The sinuses reduce the weight of the head. Sinuses also work with the voice, dealing with the range and sound that is produced.

The sinuses connect to the nasal passages of the nose, affecting the quality of breathing. If any of the sinus cavities are blocked, the ability to breathe is compromised. While excessive production of mucus can indicate infection within the membranes that line the sinus and nose, not enough can indicate congestion. Reflexology, especially working the sinus reflexes and the reflex for the nose, will assist in opening the passages, allowing the flow of mucus to be discharged or slowing down the manufacture of excess mucus.

Many people will respond with a runny nose during the session. Often these people have been very congested, even uncomfortably so. As you thumb walk along the ridge areas of the toes, you can actually see this response. This is exciting and rewarding—you are involved in helping someone feel better. Because reflexology is holistic, you are working on balancing the whole person, integrating with whatever other treatment may already be in process.

Feel the Neck and Shoulders Relax

Tension is often held in the neck and shoulders. Some people work all day at a computer, drive for long periods of time, or stand in front of a group, making a presentation. Some people carry children, lift packages, build houses, or crawl under or over spaces. Some people bend and turn and lift all day. Whatever people are doing, their necks and shoulders are involved.

The reflexes in the toes mirror the neck, and the guideline of the shoulder reflex mirrors the shoulders. Thumb walking around the entire base of the great toe affects the neck. Walking up the toes from the base also deals with the neck. The entire shoulder reflex, found on the bottom, side, and top surface of the foot, reflects the front, side, and back of the shoulders.

> • • • Reflex Points • • •
>
> Reflexologists refer to the adhesions under the skin as crystals. These crystals feel gritty and crunchy. The tiny, tight knots felt under the skin are actually a condition called tonus. Tonus is a mild spasm of muscle fibers that results in a tight, hard area that can be felt when thumb walking.

The many muscles, nerves, and blood vessels found in the neck work with the shoulders as well. Tension in the neck may generate from the shoulders, or vice versa. Often people hold their shoulders in a state of constant tension. As the shoulder muscles tighten, the neck muscles that are connected tighten as well.

As you reflex the neck and shoulder areas reflected on the foot, you may see a visible relaxation of the receiver's body. Generally, the receiver will feel warmth in the neck and shoulder region, and she may actually feel the relaxing effect begin to spread throughout her body. As the giver, you may feel the reflexes in the feet relax as well.

When you begin to reflex these areas on the feet, you may find tension, identified by hard, tight skin. The buildup of lactic acid or adhesions will often respond with a crunchy, gritty feeling. However, as you continue to reflex these areas you can truly feel a relaxation response.

Circling the Brain Reflex

The brain reflex is found on the top of all the toes. Work this reflex by thumb walking up the toe and stopping at the tip of the top. At this spot, which is one of the main reflexes for the brain, slowly begin to rotate with your thumb. As you continue to rotate on this reflex, you will feel the toe opening to the pressure from the thumb. Keep on working in the circular motion, rotating your thumb in tiny circles.

This reflex is the mirror of the main nerve center of the body, the brain, which is housed in the skull. The brain contains billions of neurons and nerve fibers and consists of many parts that receive, store, and transmit messages throughout the body, via the spinal cord.

As you circle on the brain reflex, you are connecting with the twelve pairs of cranial nerves. The nerves in the brain are either motor, sensory, or a mixture of both. These cranial nerves work with the muscles and sensory organs found in the head and neck. You are supporting the homeostasis of this organ. Keeping the brain functioning at the highest level keeps the body functioning equally as well.

PART 4

Reflexology and the Body

It's up to you to protect and maintain your body's innate capacity for health and healing by making the right choices in how you live.

—ANDREW WEIL

AT THIS POINT, you've had a chance to learn the basic techniques of reflexology, you've explored the idea of the foot as a reflection of the body, and you've discovered how to use the techniques of reflexology to help the receiver relax and reduce stress. In this part, you're going to dig further into the practice of reflexology, finding out how it relates to different body systems. The connection between reflex points of the big (great) toe and the glandular systems of the body will be covered. You'll learn where the nervous system is reflected in the foot, how to alleviate stress in the heart and lungs, how to relieve stress in the digestive system and then recharge it, how to reflex the reproductive system, and more.

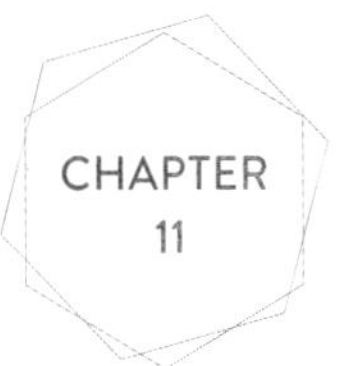

CHAPTER 11

Press This Point

The last place we tend to look for healing is within ourselves.
—WAYNE MULLER

The great toe is an important toe for walking and standing. This toe is equally as important in reflexology since it holds many reflexes for the significant glands and organs found in the head and neck. The entire great toe area holds reflex points that are integral to the proper functioning of the body. In this chapter, you'll discover the connection between the great toe and the head, including the sensory system and the endocrine system. You'll learn how various points in the toe correspond to the hypothalamus reflex, the pituitary reflex, the thyroid reflex, and more. And you'll learn which techniques to use on the foot to stimulate these glands and organs—rotation, holding, pressing, and hooking—and why it's important to do so.

Reflex Points of the Great Toe

The great toes house the reflex areas for:

- Eyes, nose, ears (and inner ears)
- Sinuses

- Mouth, throat, tongue, and teeth
- Endocrine glands of the hypothalamus, pituitary, pineal, thyroid, and parathyroid
- Brain: cerebrum, brain stem, and cerebellum

As you thumb walk, finger walk, and hook into the reflex points for the sensory organs on the great toes, you are helping the receiver maintain a state of balance within the body.

• • • Reflex Points • • •

Reflexes represent the mirrored images of the whole body linked together through zone therapy. You should not treat for a specific condition or single body part or system. Instead, work all the reflexes all the time.

The Eyes and Ears

The main reflexes for the eyes are found on both of the great toes. The right eye is on the right toe and the left eye is on the left toe. The eyes function like a camera, responding to light, acting like a shutter lens. Nerve cells in the eye receive signals from light, sending messages to the brain where the transformation of these signals into visual data occurs. Reflexology assists in the homeostasis of this operation.

The ear reflexes are also on the great toes, with supporting reflexes found elsewhere. These tiny, complex organs are very simple in design yet powerful in their functions. The ears have a broad range of responsiveness, reacting to sounds as powerful as a rocket engine or as subtle as an ocean breeze. The sounds can be near or far, yet the ears register the vibrations. Barometric pressure can affect their function pertaining to balance and the ability to assess space.

Within the ear, two other parts exist. The middle ear has three bones known as the hammer, anvil, and stirrup. These bones, named because of their shape, actually pulse with sound waves and connect with the inner ear. The inner ear has two integral functions: to send signals to the hearing center of the brain and to send signals to maintain equilibrium.

As you reflex the points that affect the function of the ears, you assist in maintaining the receiver's ability to hear clearly and to stay balanced, literally. If the receiver is suffering from blocked ears or other such symptoms, reflexology may help clear some of the congestion.

The Nose

The reflex points for the nose are reflected along the inside edge of the joints on both great toes. These bony protuberances are the guideline to find the nose reflex. As you look at both feet, placing them together, the great toes will line up and this joint will be obvious. When you thumb walk up the inside ridge of the great toe, you are moving directly into the nose reflex. As you walk up the toe from the base, you encounter a joint in the center of the great toe. Just above this joint is the nose reflex.

The nose is the transmitter of olfactory senses to the brain. The brain can identify approximately twenty thousand different scents. You are able to breathe clean air because of the filters found in the nose and nasal canal. The incredible structure of the nose allows you to filter air, transport and remove dust particles, and enjoy the beauty of scent.

• • • Reflex Points • • •

The feet are small in comparison to the body. There are many organs, glands, and other body parts represented by the reflexes that are mirror images found on the feet. Often one reflex point may overlap another, which is why you take small, tiny bites as you thumb and finger walk your way around the feet.

The Sinuses

Reflexes for the sinuses are found on all the toes, as the four other toes support the great toe. These reflexes are on the tops of the toes, along with the brain reflex. When you thumb walk up to the top of the toe, as well as walk over the toe, you are working the sinus reflex. This is a reflex where you also hold and rotate, so as to thoroughly deal with the reflection of the sinuses.

The Mouth and Throat

The mouth and throat are mirrored on the great toe, with support on the other toes. The reflexes for the mouth and throat are found along the lower inner edge of the great toe, as well as the edge at the bottom of the toe pad and the toe base.

When you thumb walk around the entire base of the toe, you are affecting the neck, half on the right and half on the left. As you thumb walk up the inner edge, just below the toe joint, you find the reflex for the mouth, teeth, and tongue. Thumb walk in and hold here for a count of three and move on up. Whenever you thumb walk along this toe edge or thumb walk the zones of the great toe, you are affecting these reflexes.

• • • Reflex Points • • •

When we refer to the inner edge of the toes or feet, it means those reflexes that are toward the inside edge of both feet. This is reflecting the midline of the body. The outer edges of the feet or toes address the reflexes nearer the outer side of the body.

The Brain

The cerebrum, the brain stem, and the cerebellum are all reflected on the great toe. The cerebrum is the frontal part of the brain with the reflexes located on the entire top of the great toe as well as the other toes. You will thumb walk over this point. Rotate, push, and hold on this reflex point.

The brain stem holds the medulla oblongata, the pons, and the midbrain. The spinal cord is a continuation of the brain stem. The reflex for this area is found on the top surface of the foot, at the base of the great toe. You will finger walk around the entire neck of the toe, affecting this reflex. You will also finger walk and thumb walk down the top surface of the toe from the tip to the base. When you work these areas, you are working the reflexes for the brain stem as well as the entire back of the head.

The cerebellum is located behind the brain stem. The reflex for the cerebellum is located on the dorsal surface of the toes, especially the great toe. This reflex and the brain stem reflex overlap. As you work on the dorsal aspect of the great toe, with finger walking and thumb walking, you are affecting areas of the brain.

The Hypothalamus Reflex

The hypothalamus is part of the endocrine system and as such deals with the chemical production in the body. This part of the brain controls many body activities and is a regulator of homeostasis. The hypothalamus is a link of integration between the endocrine and nervous systems. It deals with activities of the autonomic nervous system (ANS). It regulates the heart rate, the contractions of smooth muscle, and the movement of food through the intestinal tract.

Several hormones produced by the hypothalamus work directly with the pituitary gland. The hypothalamus is the master controller of the pituitary gland. The pituitary gland in turn influences the production of many of the hormones in the body.

This small section of the brain, the hypothalamus, is the pleasure/pain center. This area regulates your extreme feelings and your behavior regarding these emotions. This is also the area that tells you when you are hungry, when you are full, and when you are thirsty.

Even your sleep patterns have roots within the hypothalamus. Here is where your daily sleep program is established. The temperature of the flow of blood through the hypothalamus regulates your body temperature. When the blood is too hot, the ANS receives information to cool it down, and the opposite occurs if the blood is too cold. The reflex for this part of the brain is essentially the same as that of the pituitary.

The Pituitary Reflex

The pituitary reflex overlaps the hypothalamus region on the foot. You'll find this reflex on the inner edge of the great toe, just above the center joint, as shown in Figure 11.1. Thumb walk up from the base of the toe exactly along the ridge from the inside, slightly past the joint. You'll see that the toe has an indentation that receives the thumb. Once the thumb has found the reflex, rotate on the spot and hold. Turn the thumb so the side is in the actual groove. With a slight back-and-forth motion, work this reflex, moving in more deeply. As the thumb feels the reflex give, stay in this spot and press.

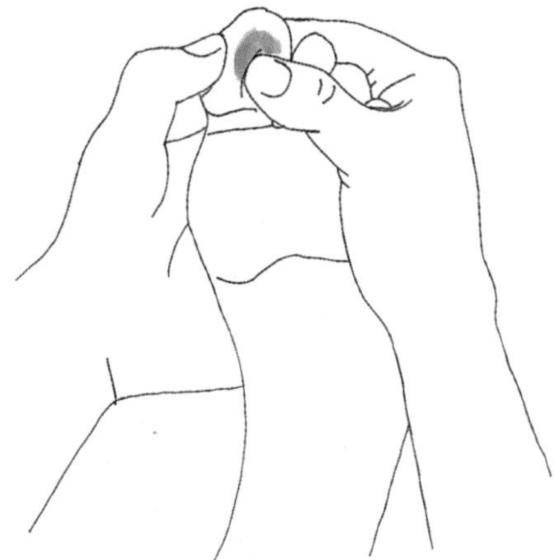

Figure 11.1 The pituitary gland reflex is on the inner ridge of the great toe.

The pituitary is pea-sized. This hormone-producing gland sits in the middle of the brain, behind the nose. It is connected to the hypothalamus, which is the governing agent. The pituitary is called the master gland, as its job is to release major hormones that will influence the entire endocrine system, in turn affecting the whole body.

Reflexology works to establish a dialogue with all parts of the body. When dealing with the pituitary gland, or any endocrine unit, the intention is to assist with homeostasis.

The Pineal Reflex

The pineal gland is a minute structure buried deep in the brain, far behind the eyes. This pinecone-shaped endocrine gland produces melatonin, which affects our sleep patterns. Sunshine helps to balance the flow and production of this hormone. Too little sun releases too much melatonin, which results in excessive sleepiness. During the winter months some people may need to find artificial sources of light to assist in keeping their hormone levels balanced.

Finding the Reflex

The reflex for the pineal gland is found in the central padded area of the great toes, directly in the center, as shown in Figure 11.2. (This reflex represents the eyes as well.) To access this reflex, first warm up the toe. This is done by thumb walking across the entire toe, up the padded area from the neck of the toe to the top. Continue to thumb walk across the toe, up and down a few times. As the thumb moves back and forth across the toe, feel the entire padded area begin to relax. Look at the toe, watching for the color to begin to change as well. At times, the pineal reflex will actually pop right out for you!

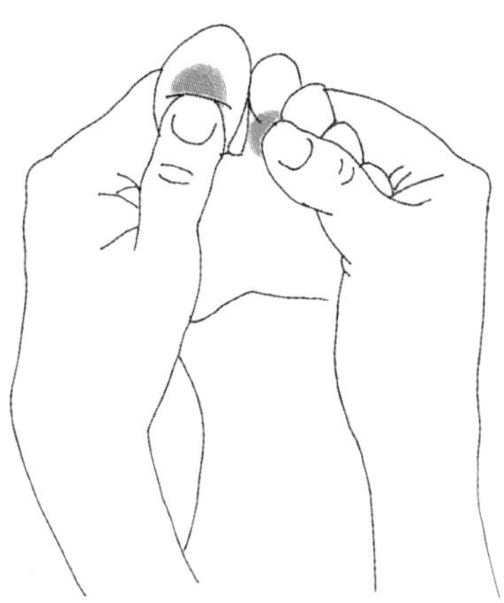

Figure 11.2 The pineal reflex is found exactly in the center of the top pad on the great toe.

Going Fishing

Above the joint line, which is in the center of the toe, thumb walk into the center of the padded area. Here, imagine X marks the spot. Place the working thumb directly on the center of that X and begin to rotate in small, steady circles. Feel the reflex as it begins to respond to you. With the thumb, circle in to the center, stop, and hold, applying even pressure. Get ready—you are going fishing now! The toe is the bait and your thumb is the fishhook. Holding the toe steady, turn the thumb on the exact reflex, push in, and hook up. The reflex may feel like a little pea under your thumb. Hold, keeping the hook in place. Working on the pineal reflex allows many receivers to reach a state of deep calm early in the session.

• • • Reflex Points • • •

Stimulation of the pineal reflex may bring about the desire for sleep in the receiver. Often when you reflex the pineal gland, the receiver will begin to relax deeply. This is a true compliment to the effectiveness of your work. Reflexology does encourage relaxation to the alpha state.

The Thyroid Reflex

The thyroid is another endocrine gland. This gland has two lobes and is found nestled in the base of the neck, just below the voice box, with a lobe on either side of the windpipe. The thyroid is shaped like a butterfly; each wing is on one side of the body.

The thyroid stores its hormones in large quantities, so the thyroid always has a supply on hand, enough to last about one hundred days. The hormones indigenous to the thyroid are thyroxine, calcitonin, and triiodothyronine. Thyroid hormones regulate oxygen use, which affects the production of heat within the body. These hormones also regulate the metabolism of the body, affecting all the processes.

Aids in Growth and Development

The thyroid gland plays an important role in the growth and development of the body. The thyroid affects the growth of nervous and muscle tissues. This gland helps to control the calcium levels, as well as reduce cholesterol. The thyroid deals with glucose conversion; glucose affects your energy level, because as glucose burns calories, more energy is produced.

Finding the Reflex

The thyroid reflex is found in the neck of the great toe, along the inside edge moving into the joint at the base of the toe. Thumb walk in toward the neck ridge, allowing the thumb to walk over the base of the toe four or five times. As you take small bites on this reflex, walk up from just below the toe neck, in at the edge, and hold. Then finger walk onto the top side of the toe at the base a few tiny steps in. The thumb also takes small circular moves along the inner edge of the toe neck.

Following these tiny moves in and around and up and down, circle on the point and hold, applying steady pressure. If there is any tightness in this area, continue to work on the reflex point. Reflexology helps move out toxins and break up congestion everywhere in the body. If the thyroid does have blockage, reflexology can help to reestablish homeostasis.

The Parathyroid Reflex

The parathyroid glands consist of two pairs, a superior and an inferior, that sit on the back of the thyroid gland. The parathyroid glands produce the hormone PTH, or parathyroid hormone. PTH deals with the balance of calcium and phosphate in the blood. Under the correct circumstance, the parathyroid hormone absorbs calcium and phosphate from the gastrointestinal (GI) tract, moving these minerals into the blood.

Calcium and Phosphate

Calcium and phosphate are structural components of bones and teeth. Phosphate works within the body structure performing a number of tasks, combining with other minerals to make DNA and RNA. Calcium is absorbed into the bloodstream and is essential for many bodily functions, including blood clotting, muscle contraction, normal heartbeat, and nerve health.

• • • Reflex Points • • •

The parathyroid also affects the kidneys. PTH speeds up the removal of calcium from the urine to the blood. At the same time, it accelerates the arrival of phosphate from the blood to the urine. Therefore, PTH increases calcium in the blood and decreases the level of phosphate in the blood.

Finding the Reflex

The reflexes for the parathyroids are found to the side and slightly under the thyroid reflex. As you look at the bottom surface of the great toe, exactly at the neck reflex, the parathyroid reflex overlaps with this reflex and the thyroid reflex as well. Thumb walk under the fat pad of the great toe right along the edge near the centerline. The second lobe reflection is found at the bottom of the thyroid reflex, along the base of the toe neck. Thumb walk in and hold, and rotate and hold, letting the thumb stay exactly on the point.

Using Rotation, Holding, Pressing, and Hooking

These techniques allow you to work deeply and more effectively, without having to apply unnecessary force. Reflexology is a loving application; every part of the session is done in honor of the receiver, to assist in his or her empowerment. As the receiver strives toward whole health, you are able to be part of the healing process.

Many areas of the feet require an assortment of thumb and finger techniques. It is important to have a working knowledge of all reflexology techniques. The feet have many bony eminences, structural hills and valleys, all of which you can and should reflex.

Rotation

Rotating on a point gives the reflexologist true access to a reflex. As the thumb circles in, the actual movement encourages the reflex to respond, letting the giver continue to move in more deeply. By staying directly on the reflex, you are continuing the communication with the area represented. Using steady, even pressure, circling in on the reflex point, continue to rotate and then hold, still allowing the point to respond. At times you can use your finger in the same fashion, on specific reflexes. For instance, when you work on the parathyroid reflex, you may use the thumb and also the index finger.

• • • Reflex Points • • •

Sometimes you will circle into a point, and as you hold steady, actually rotate the foot around the thumb. The working thumb holds on the reflex point as the holding hand turns the foot, slowly rotating in a circle. Both of these rotation movements allow you to work deeply and effectively, relieving congestion.

Holding

Holding on a point helps to clear blockage right at that point, as well as stimulate blood flow. Both the thumb and the fingers, depending upon the areas to be worked, perform this technique. Thumbs cannot always reach as effectively as the fingers. The more you practice, the better you will be able to judge this option.

Whether you thumb walk, finger walk, rotate, hook, or press onto a point, holding at the reflex supports the relaxation of that point. Maintaining even pressure allows the reflex to fully open to the work being done. Always hold on the reflex points of the brain and the endocrine points of the head.

Pressing

There are many areas during a session where pressing on a reflex is the coup de grâce. When you work on the pineal reflex after you rotate and hold, press in with your thumb and hold again. Often you will thumb walk across an area and, before moving on, press with the flat of your thumb. This is a way of sealing in the work you have just performed.

Pressing on a point or an area is a calming and reassuring way to move in deeply, without any trauma to the area or the receiver. Always work within the comfort zone of the person receiving the treatment.

Hooking

Perhaps the most advanced technique in reflexology is to hook in and pull back up. With this technique you can actually pinpoint those specific reflexes that are small and set in, representing areas deep within the body, such as the pineal gland. The hooking technique allows you to stimulate deeply in an area that is too small to effectively thumb walk within.

To apply this technique, move directly to the point and thumb press into the point. As you are pressing, begin to rotate, moving in deeper and deeper. Each circle allows a closer penetration. From this point, push into the area and hold. As you hold on the point, press in with the tip of the thumb, turn the thumb 150 degrees, push in, and pull up as though using a fishhook.

This technique allows deep penetration, yet there should be no pain, as the process is slow with steps that take the thumb into the reflex area for effective stimulation.

The key to any of these steps and points is to practice, practice, and practice. The more people you work on, the more proficient and professional you become.

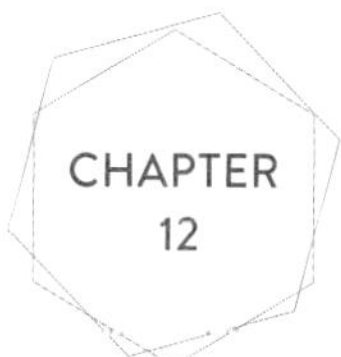

CHAPTER 12

Getting to Know the Nervous System

Seek healing, a refilling of energy and spirit, as soon as you see that you need it. You don't have to push yourself to give, do, or perform when what your body, mind, soul, and emotions need is to heal.

—MELODY BEATTIE

The nervous system and the endocrine system are in many ways the lifelines of human whole health—the keys to body, mind, and soul wellness. Reflexology connects with the central nervous system through the nerves running to and from the feet. The connection continues with the nervous system and the endocrine system through the spinal cord and the brain. In the previous chapter, you discovered the foot's connection with the endocrine system. In this chapter, the focus shifts to the spinal cord and the brain. It covers the body's need for equilibrium and explores how you as a reflexologist can help the receiver relax and reap the benefits of the practice.

The Need for Equilibrium

Homeostasis is the state of normal function for all the various systems of the body. The body is in homeostasis when the systems are responding in balance and operating at appropriate levels. The equilibrium of all body fluids, through the balance of temperature, chemical level, and internal pressure, represents good health for all cells.

You have worked with the reflex points of the head, neck, and shoulders, as well as those that deal with many of the hormone-producing glands of the endocrine system. The reflexes for the brain, the brain stem, and the sensory system are reflected in the toes you have just worked on. However, there are many compartments in the brain, and it's time to actively stimulate this network.

• • • Reflex Points • • •

The introduction of stress creates an imbalance within the environment of homeostasis. When this happens, the operating systems of the body, particularly the nervous and endocrine systems, promote a return to balance. These two systems share the maintenance of homeostasis, keeping the body functioning at a healthy level.

The Parts of the Brain

The brain has a number of different parts responsible for different functions in the body. The following are the most important:

- The **medulla oblongata** is found in the brain stem and holds the pathways of communication between the spinal cord and the various sections of the brain.
- The **pons** is the bridge that connects the spinal cord to the brain and various brain parts to each other. This part of the brain stem works with the medulla to help control respiration.
- The **midbrain** is the final piece of the brain stem. This section deals with motor and sensory nerve bundles. These nerves carry impulses from the cerebral cortex to the pons and the spinal cord. The midbrain also contains nerves that conduct energy to the thalamus.
- The **thalamus** interprets and translates sensory messages such as pain, temperature, light touch, and pressure.

- The **hypothalamus**, although small in size, conducts a major amount of business, including regulation of heart rate, digestion, flow of urine, reception of information from the internal organs, connecting the nervous system and endocrine system, and more.
- The **cerebrum** deals with the areas of sensory impulses and muscular movement as well as the areas of emotions and intellect. This center of control is divided into four sections, the lobes of the cerebrum. Each set of lobes has a specific function.
    - Frontal lobes control muscle contraction, learning ability, intellect, and emotion.
    - Parietal lobes control impulses of pain, cold, heat, touch, and pressure.
    - Temporal lobes control hearing, smell, and language development.
    - Occipital lobes control seeing, recognition of shape, color, and movement.
- The **cerebellum** is a motor region of the brain, dealing with the subconscious movements of the muscles, coordination, posture, and balance.
- The **limbic system** is the area of the brain that surrounds the brain stem and is the emotional and behavioral center, often called the "emotional brain."

Connecting the Feet, Spinal Cord, and Brain

The central nervous system (CNS) is the brain, the brain stem, and the spinal cord. The basic functional unit in the CNS is the neuron. Electrical impulses are chemically transmitted across synapses to other neurons, creating a pathway. The CNS integrates incoming information, generates thoughts and feelings, and stores memories. The impulse for muscles to contract and glands to secrete comes from the central nervous system.

The Peripheral Nervous System (PNS)

Once the neurons move into the peripheral area of the nervous system, they become nerves. The peripheral nervous system connects the CNS to sensory vehicles, muscles, and glands. The peripheral nervous system is composed of cranial and spinal nerves. These nerves carry information in and out of the central nervous system. Sensory neurons carry information from sensory receptors in the body into the CNS, while motor neurons carry impulses out of the CNS to the muscles and glands.

Somatic and Autonomic Nervous Systems

The peripheral system can be further divided into the somatic and autonomic nervous systems. The somatic nervous system (SNS) carries information from sensory receptors in the head, body frame, and limbs to the brain. Information dealing with movement travels from the brain via motor receptors to skeletal muscles. The autonomic nervous system (ANS) conveys sensory information from the organs to the CNS, while motor neurons carry information from the brain to smooth muscle, glands, and the heart muscle.

Spinal Nerve

The nerves of the spinal cord connect the central nervous system to the operations of the body. Remember, these nerves are part of the peripheral nervous system. There are thirty-one pairs of spinal nerves emerging out of the bones that house the spinal cord. (The bones form a column called the vertebral column.) These nerves travel out over the entire body, connecting with all the operating systems.

One branch of the nerves found in the feet stems from the largest nerve in our body, the sciatic nerve. The sciatic nerve sends its two branches down the leg into the foot. In the foot these nerves branch out again, with many divisions serving the entire area.

7,200 Nerve Endings

Nerves are excitable tissue, covered and protected by connective tissue. Blood vessels within these coverings feed the nerves. Spinal nerves are mixed nerves containing both sensory and motor impulses. Skeletal muscles receive motor stimulation from neurons within spinal nerves. What is most important to understand is that the feet contain many nerves, providing signals throughout the body, as well as receiving signals from outside stimuli.

• • • Reflex Points • • •

Reflex response can be simple or complex, depending upon the nerves involved. Simple reflexes involve one sensory and one motor neuron, while complex reflexes involve a relationship with more than two neurons. For example, the stretch reflex is simple, and the tendon reflex is complex.

Seeing the Receiver Relax

As a reflexologist you become aware that each segment of the session provokes a deeper relaxation response in the receiver. From the moment of arrival, the receiver has begun the process of de-stressing. For some people, just the thought of returning for treatment is often enough to activate the relaxation reaction. As you study this technique you will learn to pick up cues from the receiver. As the receiver is made comfortable, you allow the receiver the right to relax. Your first words relay the message. For many receivers the permission to relax and let go is essential.

• • • Reflex Points • • •

Trust is essential in this process. The receiver must feel safe and secure from the beginning of the session. The giver establishes an environment of caring through firm, gentle touch. A quiet, clean ambiance is important; a compassionate, genuine treatment is vital.

The next important piece in this process is the introduction of touch. The relaxation techniques facilitate relaxation of the feet as well as of the body and of the mind. By accessing the nervous system through steady, even touch, the receiver is able to truly relax and trust.

Moving on from the relaxation segment, you begin to finger walk the toes. Stay focused on the receiver, being aware of the pressure used as well as the routine. The face of the receiver is easily read; the more relaxed the person becomes, the harder it will be for his eyes to stay open. The color of the skin will respond, beginning to display a healthy glow.

Alpha is a meditative state that is often entered into through deep relaxation. Freedom from stress brings more relaxed breathing; the receiver generally releases deep sighs signaling a tranquil state. Make sure you have a light cover over the person you are working on, as the body temperature does drop.

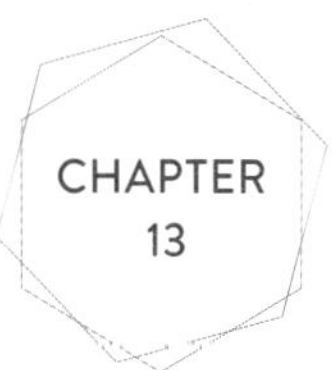

CHAPTER
13

Warm the Heart from the Sole

In dwelling, be close to the land. In meditation, go deep in the heart.
In dealing with others, be gentle and kind.

—LAO TZU

Close your eyes for a moment and picture your body. What organs and parts of the body reside in the area from the shoulder guideline to the diaphragm guideline? Did you picture your heart and lungs? Those are the organs that will be reflected in this stage of a reflexology session. In this chapter, you'll learn how to use basic techniques you've already learned, such as the knuckle press and thumb walk, to relieve stress in this area by focusing on the corresponding zone in the foot. Don't forget the top surface—all parts of the foot need attention!

The Ball of the Foot

This area of the foot is part of the forefoot, housing the metatarsal heads and top halves of the five metatarsal bones. The fleshy section of the ball is located under the joints that bend the toes at their base. This top sector of the ball of the foot contains the metatarsal heads, and the rest of the ball holds the long metatarsal bones. Various muscles, tendons, and ligaments work to hold the bones together.

Let your fingers trace the top of the foot, and you will feel the metatarsals. The first bone is short and wide, and the other four are thin and long. Look at the sole now and see how the entire ball of the foot puffs out, just like the chest region of the body.

• • • Reflex Points • • •

The ball of the foot is the area that we spring off of when we walk. There is a point during the cycle of walking where the forefoot bears all of the body weight. These tiny bones do a tremendous amount of work! Often people will have calluses, dry skin, even pinched nerves due to improper shoe gear and walking habits.

If you pull the top of the foot down toward the sole, a natural line will appear under the ball of the foot, which is the diaphragm line. The entire region from under the toes, which is the shoulder line, to this line in the arch is the area we are dealing with now.

This part of the foot holds reflexes for the heart, lungs, trachea, bronchioles, breast, some of the skeletal system, and the upper back. The reflex for the thymus gland is found here as well as the reflexes of the lymphatic system. The areas of representation are fairly straightforward, although some regions do overlap. For the most part, the locations of the reflexes are exactly where you would imagine them to be.

Begin with a Knuckle Press

Working on the right foot and holding with your left hand, prepare to continue on with this section. Your right hand will form a closed fist as you use the outside of the long bones to press into the foot. With your left hand solidly behind the foot, your hand is acting like a cup, letting the fingers provide the support. Another option is to firmly grasp the toes with the left hand, holding the foot straight and tall, as you press into this section of the foot.

Establish a Rhythm

Support the foot as you gently and firmly press into the entire ball of the foot. Begin with the top region of this area and press down and up continuously for a number of presses. Look at the face of the receiver; encourage him to relax and breathe deeply. This is a relaxing technique that can be used throughout the session, whenever you feel the need for transitional assistance.

Continue to press in and let your body move gently, establishing a rhythm. Press in as you move in. Let the fist rock a bit on the foot, flowing from knuckles to finger joints and back to knuckles again.

• • • Reflex Points • • •

Never push in deeply. The foot will open to your pressure as you work. Even if the receiver wants you to push harder, explain you are working at the right level at this time. Trust that when the body is ready, you will have deeper access.

Think of Kneading

Another way to describe the knuckle press is to equate this technique to the motion of kneading. Kneading the ball of the foot is connecting you with all the reflexes found in the chest region. As you knead, let the supporting hand press in on the top of the foot, keeping the rhythm. This provides a comforting feeling to the person receiving the treatment.

The knuckle press is a good technique for large areas of the foot that may have tougher skin, like the ball and the heel. This does not mean you can push heavily! If anything, you need to be more sensitive since the knuckles have no feeling. You need to be aware of how deeply you are pressing, adjusting to the receiver's comfort zone.

Thumb Walk the Heart Reflex

Now that you have relaxed the chest region, you are ready to move on. Place both feet together for a moment so you can see the relationship of the heart reflex in the feet to that of the position of the heart in the body. Look at the shape of the feet and notice how the swell of the ball is greater on the inside edges of the feet, especially at the base. This reflects the heart; the base of the ball of the foot located at the inner edge is the heart reflex.

Use the left hand to press on the right foot while the right hand supports the foot. When working this area on the left foot, switch hands. Doing this frees up each hand, allowing the thumbs the ability to work without strain.

Finding the Reflex

Use the knuckle press again to create the flow, and after a few presses, let the second joint of your index finger trace a line. This line will run from the bottom base at the outside edge of the great toe down around the whole metatarsal head, which seems like a continuation of the great toe. Look at the foot again. See the slight crease, or indentation, that runs from the great toe down to the diaphragm line? This is the line you glide your second joint over. Let the joint glide around and down, and the reflex will pop right out. This is the heart reflex, with more on the left side than on the right. You will actually see the skin peek out a bit from the side of the foot.

• • • Reflex Points • • •

If the receiver has any circulatory issues, such as high blood pressure, or is on any kind of heart medication, use an alternative technique. Using the left thumb, thumb walk across the diaphragm line from the outside edge of the foot to the inner edge. The heart reflex will still pop right out.

Working the Reflex

Now that you have located the heart reflex, gently use the thumb of the supporting hand to circle on the reflex. The supporting hand is still holding the foot; the thumb is brought to the side to perform the circling technique. Let the thumb softly and slowly circle on this reflex, and soon the area will feel warm.

After making small circles, thumb walk over the reflex as well. Here the thumb of the supporting hand is still doing the walking; essentially, both thumbs have met at the heart. Thumb walk from many different angles on this reflex point, coming in from all sides in small, steady bites. Finish this reflex with small circles and a gentle stroking off.

Caterpillar the Chest Reflex Region

Let the left hand support the foot again, as the right hand will start the sequence. Using the right thumb, you are going to thumb walk the chest region in an inchworm, or caterpillar, type movement.

Beginning at the heart reflex, thumb walk up from the heart reflex to under the great toe, turn, and thumb walk down to the diaphragm line. Continue to thumb walk in this manner up to the base of the toes and down to the diaphragm line in a curvy line until the thumb reaches the outside edge of the foot. The left hand is holding the foot, gently clasping the toes, as the right thumb walks across the reflexes. The fingers of your right hand may rest on the top surface of the foot while the thumb does the work.

• • • Reflex Points • • •

This caterpillar technique is the preliminary walk-through for all the reflexes on the ball of the foot. Each little bite is working on reflexes that deal with the lungs, windpipe, bronchi, bronchioles, breasts, upper lymphatics, thymus, or the heart. Each foot contains the same reflexes.

Do not overstretch your hand. If you feel the thumb is pulling away from the fingers, curl the fingers up behind the thumb; the fingers come along for the ride as the thumb works across the ball of the foot. There will be many times throughout a session where you will need to adapt your reach. Always pay attention to your form; if you feel your fingers stretching away from one another, readjust.

Once the right thumb has created the curvy path from the inside edge to the outer edge, switch hands. Now the right hand is the supporting hand and the left hand is the one doing the work. Use the left thumb to caterpillar back across the ball of the foot. Take small bites, turning down into the curves each time and walking up again. This movement will bring you back to the heart reflex again.

Thumb Walk from the Inside Edge

Use the left hand to support the foot, either by holding the toes or holding the foot firmly. The right hand is the working hand. Return to the heart reflex and prepare to thumb walk. Look at the foot for a moment, visualizing what you are getting ready to do. Imagine the two guidelines you are working between, the shoulder line and the diaphragm line. Notice how this section of the foot is shaped, almost rectangular. The two edges of the foot would be the sides, and the guidelines are the top and bottom, creating a rectangle. The heart reflex is located in the bottom right of this rectangular box.

Thumb walk along the diaphragm line from the heart reflex. Stop just over the central tendon line, which is right in the reflex point for the bronchioles. Quickly and smoothly bring the thumb back to the heart reflex. Move the thumb up just a bit above the heart reflex point and thumb walk in again just beyond the tendon line. The reflexes for the bronchioles and bronchi begin to overlap.

As you continue to move up this section of the foot, you are working on the lungs and bronchioles. Always thumb walk slowly to the center and bring the thumb back to the inner edge of the foot to follow the next line up. Each line up this side of the ball is working toward the shoulder line. Imagine that this process is like stacking sheets of paper in one side of a rectangular box, continuing to stack until this side is full.

Just before the shoulder line, at the very top edge of the first metatarsal, close to the inner side, is the thymus reflex. Begin by thumb walking the line to the center and bring the thumb back, to rest on the reflex point for the thymus. Place the thumb directly under the shoulder line, just below the neck and thyroid reflex, along that inner edge.

The reflex may or may not feel a bit bony or bumpy under the thumb. Regardless, this is the thymus reflex. Rotate the thumb on this point. Feel the reflex relax under the thumb as you rotate in small circles. Stop and hold on this point, pressing down gently on the reflex.

Once you have completed thumb walking up this portion of the rectangle, you will thumb walk down in the same fashion. Starting from the thymus reflex, thumb walk in to the center and bring the thumb back to the edge, just under the thymus point. Continue to walk down this side of the ball of the foot, until the last swipe across comes from the diaphragm line. You will now move over to the left side of this section of the foot.

Thumb Walk from the Outside Edge

The essence of the work here is to complete the other side of the rectangular box that you have created over the ball of the foot. The right hand is now the supporting hand, and the left hand has become the working hand. The routine for the reflexes on the ball of the foot is the same on both feet. Begin with the left thumb on the outer edge of the diaphragm line; this will be the left edge of the foot as you look at it.

Thumb walk with slow, small steps to the tendon line, then bring the thumb back to the outer edge. Continue to thumb walk into the center, each time moving the thumb up a bit to create a new line from the outer edge. Again, imagine stacking sheets of paper on top of one another to build the other piece of the rectangle.

As you thumb walk over this region you continue to work on the lung reflex. Reflexology promotes circulation, and working on reflexes signals the muscles of the body to let go and relax. When the lung region releases tension, the entire chest area settles down and accepts the healing. Often the receiver will cough or sigh, a signal that tension is leaving.

By walking in and out of this side of the chest region, you are also working the breast reflex. Thumb walk the breast reflex and continue up the foot, walking in toward the tendon line and coming back out to the edge of the foot to start a new line. At the shoulder line, repeat the process, moving down the foot to the diaphragm line.

• • • Reflex Points • • •

The dorsal (top) surface of the foot reflects the back of the body, and the sole reflects the front. Many reflexology foot charts place the breast reflex on the top of the foot. Perhaps this placement mirrors components of the lymphatic system. However, for our purposes, the breast reflex mirrors the breast location on the body.

Butterfly the Area

The butterfly technique is a wonderful transitional move. Cup the foot in both hands, with one hand on each side of the foot. Remember to rest the fingers of both hands on the top surface of the foot, allowing the thumbs freedom of movement. The thumbs will walk along the plantar surface, in this case from the shoulder line to the diaphragm line. The thumbs work together, taking small, tiny steps moving toward the centerline of the foot.

• • • Reflex Points • • •

Making a proper transition from one section to another, or from one technique to another, is easily attained with this technique. The butterfly movement signals two types of transitions. First, you are leaving the bottom surface and moving to the top for the next segment. Second, you will be using a different technique on the dorsal surface.

Start at the edge of the foot, with the thumbs at the shoulder line. Imagine for a moment the wings of a butterfly superimposed on the ball of the foot. Let the thumbs begin to walk the faint lines that represent the pattern of the wings. As the thumbs reach the center of the foot, bring the thumbs back to the edge and move down a thumb length. Both thumbs are resting on the sides of the foot. Move down a bit and walk in again to the centerline. The tendon that runs down the middle of the plantar surface of the foot divides the foot in half. Continue to butterfly in to the center, bring the thumbs back to the sides, and repeat. When the thumbs reach the diaphragm line, work back up the foot using the same process.

With this butterfly technique all of the reflexes are affected. By working in this manner you ensure that every point has been reflexed—that nothing has been overlooked. The beauty of reflexology is that many reflex points do overlap; therefore, a technique like the butterfly allows you to effectively contact all areas.

Work On the Top Surface of the Foot

The top of the foot represents the back area of the body. There are two divisions, using the diaphragm line to create the separation. Picture your back. Imagine a line representing the actual diaphragm muscle, this will be the line that divides the back into upper and lower regions. The back of the body consists of major muscles and bones, along with the spine. Place both feet together to picture what is represented here.

What's in a Back?

Sit and look at the tops of your own feet. Get comfortable and imagine the back of your body mirrored on your feet. The inner edge of both feet represents the spine. The imaginary guideline of the shoulder represents the shoulder. The two feet house reflexes for all bones and muscles of both the upper and lower back.

For this section, you are concerned only with the upper-back reflection. In this upper region of the foot are reflexes for the scapula, which is commonly known as the shoulder blade. The reflex points for the muscles that attach to this bone—the trapezius, the rhomboids, and the levator scapulae—are reflected in this area as well. The reflex for the rib cage is also represented here.

Try the Technique

The foot will rest comfortably as you position both hands on either side of the foot, at the thoracic region. Rest the thumbs on the plantar surface; they will provide leverage. Begin a slow, steady, even finger walk, with all fingers moving together toward the center of the foot. This movement seems as though the fingers are crawling together. Imagine the foot is an accordion; you are playing the notes as your fingers move in between each long metatarsal bone. Keep finger walking until the fingers meet; the fingernails will actually click together, signaling that the fingers cannot move any farther.

• • • Reflex Points • • •

This technique could generate heat in the back area of the body. The receiver may relate an extreme feeling of relaxation and be able to let go of the tension held in the back and neck.

Slowly walk the fingers back, letting the fingers inch backward. This is done exactly as it sounds. From the center, pull all the bent fingers back a bit, then straighten out the fingers slightly and then go right back onto the tips again. Let the fingers drag slightly. Picture walking between the ribs as the fingers move across the bones.

You are not digging in here, nor are you applying pressure to this bony area. Instead you are inching back, holding, pressing, and inching back again. Continue until both hands reach the edges of the foot.

Full-Finger Walking

The fingers are resting on the sides of the foot, waiting for you to make the next move. Keeping the thumbs on the bottom of the foot, again for leverage, move all the fingers up to just under the toe neck. Tuck the fingers into the little shelf created by the joints that bend the toes in that region. The tips of the fingers are touching and the fingers are flexed, ready to move.

Using all of the fingers at once, slowly finger walk down the top surface of the foot, inching along. Keep an eye on the imaginary guideline. When the fingers reach the diaphragm line, stop. Hold the fingers here, apply light pressure, and with a slight side-to side, squiggly motion, pull back to the base of the toes. Finger walk back down and repeat.

All of the upper-back reflexes receive attention with this two-part technique. You have sent communication supporting the delivery of oxygen and blood to the back area of the body. If any toxic buildup is present, the reflexology will assist in releasing this tension.

Lymph Drainage

To review, there are several major components of the lymphatic system. The fluid is called lymph and is transported by the lymphatic vessels. The lymph passes from the vessels through lymph nodes back into vessels and continues on throughout the body in this fashion. Certain organs also have lymphatic tissue: the spleen, the thymus, and the tonsils. Lymph is one of the main defense systems of the body, providing resistance to invaders. Lymph drainage is important, as it allows the flow of lymph to continue unobstructed.

The technique for lymph drainage is simple. Both feet have the same reflexes. You are still on the right foot. The thumb and forefinger are used simultaneously for this movement.

Begin with a practice run on your hands. Use your right hand to work on your left. Turn the left hand so that the palm is facing you; the thumb will be closest to you. Place your right thumb at the top of the web between the thumb and forefinger of the left hand, on the palm's surface. Rest your index finger at the top of the web, on the dorsal surface of the hand. Press in gently, feeling contact. Curl the remaining fingers into a fist, so they stay out of the way and can easily move with you.

Using slow, steady movement, inch forward and allow the thumb and finger to walk down the web toward the wrist. When you have gone as far as your hand will allow, press and hold. Gently, with light, even pressure, slowly pull back along the route you just traveled. When the two fingers reach the top of the web, hold and press the two fingers together at the tips, through the web. Gently pull off and move to the next space between the fingers, repeating to the end and back again.

• • • Reflex Points • • •

Sometimes the hands are too small to use both fingers together. If this is the case, walk down the top surface and pull back, and then walk down the bottom surface. Repeat for each web.

Now, move to the foot. The left hand is supporting the right foot, holding at the heel. Place the right thumb and forefinger at the web between the great toe and second toe. The thumb is touching the plantar surface, and the forefinger is on the dorsal side. Close the remaining fingers into a fist, tucked out of the way.

Thumb and finger walk down the foot toward the ankle. Again go as far as your hand will allow. At the end of each walk down, before moving to the next web, gently pull up to the top again. The pressure is steady, but not heavy.

Solar Plexus Reflex

The solar plexus reflex is found directly in the center of the foot, just under the diaphragm line, as shown in Figure 13.1. A plexus is a meeting place for a group of nerves, a vital center of activity. This network in turn relates to specific areas and organs in the body. As part of the autonomic nervous system, the solar plexus has sympathetic and parasympathetic nerve cells.

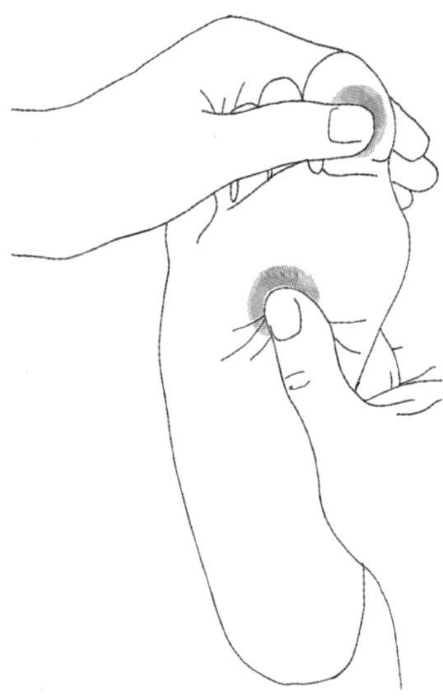

Figure 13.1 The solar plexus reflex is directly in the center of the foot just under the diaphragm line.

Solar Plexus Reflex Connections

The solar plexus seems to be related to emotional and spiritual issues. The physical organs close to this region are the diaphragm, breasts, heart, and lungs. Its name implies the power of its function. You work on the sole to treat the soul; the solar plexus is the key.

This is perhaps the most singularly powerful reflex, providing relief from painful points, as well as having a strong connection to breath. The solar plexus reflex relates to the nervous system, assisting in overall relaxation.

Working the Reflex

This reflex is the same on both feet, though you are working on the right foot at the moment. Cradle the right foot with the left hand; pull the toes down over the shoulder line, and an indentation will appear exactly at the center just below the diaphragm line. This point is aligned in zones two and three and is the beginning of the kidney meridian. Holding the foot steady, the right thumb walks in from the medial edge along the diaphragm line to the point directly under the center at the ball of the foot.

Using the entire flat surface of the thumb, turn the finger slightly sideways, pressing into the depression to identify the reflex. While the right thumb is pressing into the reflex, use the left hand to pull down from the top of the foot, effectively creating an awning over the reflex. Hold here and ask the receiver to breathe in deeply, holding the breath for a count of three and then slowly releasing.

• • • Reflex Points • • •

This technique will often release congestion felt in other reflexes. As you work, if a reflex is painful, use the solar plexus method to reduce this response. Often, activating the solar plexus is enough to reduce or eliminate the painful response.

As the receiver relaxes, release the toes while continuing to press the thumb into the reflex. At times the reflex will actually pulse, which is a signal that the reflex is involved with the sense of calmness spreading through the body. Slowly back the thumb out of the reflex, feeling the skin push up against the thumb. This technique is very effective, creating an immediate relaxation response.

Flutter Off

At the end of this section, use the flutter movement. Place both hands on the top of the foot. Using soft, fluttery strokes, move the fingers up and off the foot. The stroke is performed by gently moving the fingers on the surface of the foot. Act as though the foot is a piano keyboard, with all fingers playing at once, moving up toward the ankle.

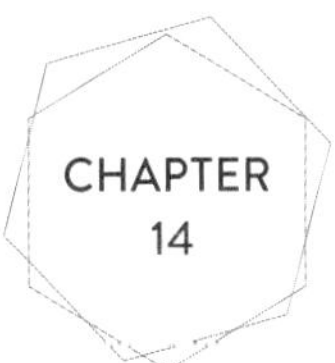

Reflexology and the Digestive System

When you make peace with yourself, you make peace with the world.
—*MAHA GHOSANANDA*

By now you are probably seeing how reflexology can help others. You have learned to relax people just by the way you touch their feet. Perhaps you have witnessed a stuffy nose run or an achy shoulder feel less tense. Whatever outcomes you have observed, you have more amazing routines to learn. In this chapter, you'll take a trip through the alimentary canal—the digestive system—and learn how to use reflexology to relieve stress in this part of the body. You'll use the same basic techniques you learned before, but you'll be applying them in new ways.

Diaphragm Line to Waistline

Remember, you're still working on the right foot. After the warm-up, always complete the routine on the right foot before moving to the left. Look at the sole of the foot and trace the diaphragm line, which runs from the outside edge of the foot to the inside edge, right along the fold of the ball of the foot. Remember, this is where the chest reflexes end. Now look at the inside edge of the great toe from just above the base, where the ridge from the second joint bulges out. This is the beginning of the esophagus reflex. Trace that down for a moment, to just below the diaphragm line, along the inside edge. The esophagus reflex will flow into the stomach reflex.

The Middle of the Arch

You are looking at the section of the foot between the diaphragm line and the waistline. Both sides of the foot represent the lines to create a new box, a rectangular shape that will hold the reflexes between the diaphragm line and the waistline guideline. The waistline coincides with the center of the foot, in the middle of the arch. Follow the little toe down into the fifth metatarsal; this long bone actually ends with a slight protuberance along the outside of the foot. Place your finger or thumb across the sole coming from this bone. Notice how the thumb is almost exactly in the middle of the arch.

Picture What Corresponds in the Body

You will be working on the reflex for the mouth and esophagus first. The mouth reflex is found on both toes just above the bottom inside edge of the toe bone. The reflex for the esophagus runs along the medial edge from the bulge of the bone along the inner edge to just below the diaphragm line. The esophagus moves right into the stomach reflex.

Look at both feet and imagine that part of your body from the diaphragm to the waist. This is the upper abdominal area, housing many organs and structures. Rest your hands on this area of your body; your thumbs naturally rest on the edges of your ribs as your fingertips touch in the center. A strong casing of muscles protects the organs within. The stomach is the next organ you encounter. The stomach is J-shaped, with most of the fatty part of the letter in the left upper portion of the abdomen. The reflex for the stomach is reflected on both feet.

The lower portion of the stomach moves toward the intestines. A valve at the end of the stomach, known as the pyloric sphincter, keeps the processed food from reentering the stomach. The reflex for the pyloric sphincter is found only on the right foot.

The Deep Organs

Picture the deeper organs that sit behind or below the stomach. The pancreas lies behind the stomach and, like the stomach, connects with the small intestine. The liver lies completely on the right side of the body, and the gallbladder is tucked in under the liver. The stomach, pancreas, liver, and gallbladder all empty into the duodenum, the piece of the intestines that connects with the pyloric sphincter just about right of the center of the waistline.

• • • Reflex Points • • •

Remember, reflexes are not body parts. A reflex is a point that energetically reflects the area of the body that it represents. One way reflexology connects to areas of the body is through the nervous system. When you reflex points you are sending energetic and electric messages to encourage homeostasis.

The reflexes for these organs or structures are reflected on the coinciding feet. The liver and gallbladder are only on the right foot, whereas the pancreas is on both feet, just as in the body. The duodenum is found on the right foot.

Another organ that is found in the upper abdomen is the spleen. The reflex for the spleen is found only on the left foot, tucked under the outer ledge of the sole, along the diaphragm line.

The adrenal glands sit on top of the kidneys, one on each side of the body, behind the liver and the stomach, tucked up under the last set of ribs. The reflexes for the adrenal glands are found just above the waistline guideline in the center of each foot.

The Middle Back

Think about your middle back, the area that begins just below your shoulder blades and ends at your waist. The ribs and the muscles that cover the ribs form the midback region of the body. These protect the inner organs and the spinal column. Many people have back pain in this region often from improper standing, sitting, and walking. Of course, for some people the pain may be generated through repetitive movement. The reflexes for this section of the body are found on the top of the foot, from just below the toes to the center of the top where the metatarsals end.

The Lower Back

The back continues down into the sacral and coccyx region of the body. In reflexology, this section of the body is represented on the dorsal surface of the foot and again when you work with the spine reflex. If you continue on the top of the foot when you are working the middle-back reflex, you will walk right on into the lower-back reflex. This brings you to the bones behind the metatarsals just in front of the ankle.

Thumb Walk the Esophageal Reflex

Working on the right foot, begin by holding the foot with your right hand, using your left hand to perform the first sequence. The right hand cradles the foot for support and leverage.

Working the Reflex

Bring the left thumb to the inner, lower edge of the great toe, just above the second joint. This is the mouth reflex. Position the thumb so it is facing down and rotate on the reflex. Rotate in a circular motion, press, and hold. Very slowly, using a firm, gentle touch, thumb walk down the inner edge of the foot, from the great toe. Thumb walk over the medial edge of the metatarsal head moving down the foot. This area may feel like a bony ridge or may have a little padding, depending on the shape of the foot. The thumb is walking on the exact medial edge; this is the reflex for the esophageal tube.

Continue thumb walking down this edge past the metatarsal head to just below the diaphragm line. Bring the thumb back up and walk down again. Feel how the reflex begins to relax under the thumb.

• • • Reflex Points • • •

Try this move on yourself. Thumb walk along this reflex and see how your foot feels. Are there any tender spots; do you need to ease up the pressure? This is a great way to find out how your technique feels—always try any of the segments that are possible on your own feet.

Three Fingers Mark the Spot

The left hand is the holding hand. Hold the right foot by the toes or cradle the foot in the palm. The left hand will provide support and stability as well as leverage. Look at the plantar surface of the foot, visualizing the two guidelines. Find the centerline of the foot and place your first three fingers to this line from the inside edge of the foot. The fingers look like three stacks of wood piled up, one on top of the other.

When holding the fingers to the centerline, the second knuckles seem to rest at the inner edge of the foot. The index finger is lying on the waistline, the middle finger is lying just above the index finger, and the ring finger is lying just under the diaphragm line. These fingers are holding the place of three reflexes, marking the spot.

Proceed with Thumb Walking

Now remove the fingers. Beginning at the top area, where the ring finger was, thumb walk slowly across this line to the center mark. Feel the foot under your thumb as it begins to relax, as the reflex responds to the pressure. Thumb walk along the next reflex, that of the pancreas. Move slowly, taking tiny bites as the thumb walks in toward the centerline of the foot. Thumb walk the last line, which is the reflex for the duodenum. Again, using small, slow moves, let the thumb walk along this reflex into the tendon line.

Bring your thumb to the end of the waistline at the inner edge of the foot, the outside edge of the duodenum reflex. Turn the thumb and walk up in a straight line to the diaphragm line. Bring the thumb back, moving in a bit along the waistline, and thumb walk up again to the diaphragm line. Repeat this movement until the thumb reaches the centerline.

Switch Hands

Switch hands and use the right hand to hold the foot while the left thumb walks from the centerline out along the reflex for the stomach. Bring the left thumb back to the tendon line and thumb walk along the pancreas reflex out to the inside edge of the foot. Lastly, thumb walk along the waistline from the center of the foot to the inner edge, reflexing the duodenum reflex. Switch hands again and, using the right thumb, repeat the thumb-walking technique from the inner edge of the foot to the centerline for the three reflexes. Walk each one slowly, feeling how the area has changed under your thumb.

• • • Reflex Points • • •

When you move back to an area already worked, you'll likely see that the initial stiffness or tightness has disappeared; the area is much more giving now. It's as though the foot has let its guard down, trusting you. This is body wisdom, recognizing the reflexology as a good thing.

Liver and Gallbladder Reflexes

The liver and gallbladder reflexes are easy to find. Place the three fingers back across the areas you have just worked. The area of the foot still showing is the liver reflex. Yes, it is that big; don't forget that the liver is the largest gland in the body. Notice how the area is shaped a bit like a slanted triangle, with the point tucked under the breast reflex. The reflex stretches over behind the stomach reflex and down to just below the guideline for the waist, along the outside edge of the foot.

Don't take those fingers away yet. Using the middle finger as a guideline, place your left thumb one joint in from the outside edge, in line with that finger. Press in slightly, feeling the depression; this is the gallbladder reflex!

Walk the Reflex

Support the foot with the right hand. Use the left thumb to walk over the entire liver reflex. This is done by thumb walking each section, bringing the thumb back to the outside edge of the foot, then moving along the next section. Walk the reflex completely, from the edge in.

Now bring the thumb to the corner of the waistline guide, along the outside edge. Turn the thumb toward the diaphragm line and walk up the reflex. Keep bringing the thumb back to the waist guideline and, each time, move in a bit toward the center before walking up again. These two moves look like you have just created a grid of lines, sideways and up, crossing over one another.

Move your thumb back to the gallbladder reflex. Let your thumb drop right into this recess and rotate on the point. As you feel the thumb moving in deeper, hook into the reflex. Hook here by pressing in and pulling the thumb back toward the edge of the foot, while still in the reflex. Hold on this point, waiting to feel the gentle give of the reflex, then release.

Be Gentle

This area is often a tender spot for people. The tenderness could be the entire liver reflex or the gallbladder reflex or both. Be aware and remind the receiver to tell you if the pressure is too hard or the reflex is too painful.

The reason for the pain may be any number of causes. It is not your job to identify why the area is painful. Rather, it is your job to continue to work within the comfort level of the receiver. If the question does arise, simply state that you do not know why it is painful and move on, advising the person to speak to his medical team about it.

Spleen Reflex

You are moving into areas where the reflexes are different on the two feet. Until now, the sequence has been the same, as the reflection of the body is similar. With the introduction of this section, however, you will see the divisions. The spleen reflex is found in the far left corner of the left foot, tucked under the outside end of the diaphragm guideline. This reflex is on the plantar surface of the foot and is fairly easy to identify.

Although you are not finished with the right foot, look at the left foot for a moment. Hold this foot in your left hand; the spleen reflex is accessed with the right thumb. Remind yourself of the diaphragm guideline, and as you do so, place your thumb one digit in from the outside edge, just under the line. Interestingly, the thumb will drop into a dip here, as there is a slight giving of the tension of the skin at this point.

Press the thumb into the reflex and hold. Firmly rotate on this spot, feeling the thumb move in deeper. As the reflex relaxes, hold the thumb on this spot, press, and hook back toward the edge of the foot. Allow the thumb to stay in the reflex, holding the hook in place.

This is another reflex that may be sensitive. The area of the foot where the spleen reflex is located is part of the lateral column. This is the section of the foot that is used for support, which could cause tenderness. Again, it is not your job to find the cause of the tenderness; you just need to be aware of it and continue on.

Gallbladder Meridian

Rest the left foot for now, covered and relaxed, and go back to the right foot. The gallbladder reflex, which is tucked up under the liver reflex, has another access point. The gallbladder meridian is one of the meridians that travels through almost the entire body. This meridian begins in the head, at the outside corner of the eye. It moves up into the head in a meandering pattern, covering a large area on the side of the head. Imagine holding the sides of your head with both hands; this is similar to the pattern and area covered by the meridian.

The meridian continues flowing down the body in this zigzag manner, branching in at the diaphragm, waist, groin, and hip. From the hip this meridian travels through the leg and knee, close to the lateral edge. The gallbladder meridian ends at the fourth toe, with the line coming across the surface of the foot.

Here is where it gets really interesting. The gallbladder reflex is one thumb joint in from the lateral edge of the right foot. The gallbladder meridian line runs right through this reflex to terminate at the fourth toe. Here is a clear joining of two modalities, connecting with the same organ. The meridian shows a pathway of energy that when blocked may cause certain disorders. The physical gallbladder helps with digestion and the energetic pathway deals with keeping the process clear.

Don't Forget the Adrenals

You are working on the right foot at the moment. Place those three fingers of the right hand back onto the reflexes that represent the adrenals. The finger you are interested in is the index finger, which is resting on the waistline guide. The padded section of the first joint in this finger is resting on the adrenal reflex and a portion of the kidney reflex as well.

The left hand is holding the foot, with the thumb resting on the sole, ready to move. Using the left thumb, walk along the waistline from the outside edge of the foot. Keep thumb walking right under the index finger, so that the tip of the finger is resting at the edge of the thumbnail bed. Remove the index finger, move the thumb up a bit toward the diaphragm line, then pull the thumb back slightly; this is the adrenal reflex.

• • • Reflex Points • • •

Don't be discouraged if at first you do not feel the pushing back or letting go that often comes with the release in a reflex. The release is happening whether you feel the slight change or not. As you practice and trust your work, you, too, will feel the giving of the reflex.

Another way to check the location of this point is to line up under the solar plexus reflex (see Chapter 13). The adrenal reflex and the solar plexus reflex are not in a straight connecting line; the adrenal may be a bit more toward the inner side of the foot, along the tendon line. Whichever way you choose to find this reflex point, when you think you have found it, rotate on the spot. You will feel a slight swell or bump on the reflex, indicating you have found the point.

Continue to rotate on the adrenal reflex, applying light pressure. When working on the adrenal reflexes, use a gentle touch, with no undue pressing. Now hold on the spot while gently pressing in. The reflex may push back, indicating it is time to move on.

Finish with Four-Finger Walking

Move to the top of the foot now. Imagine the entire back, as this is the area of reflection you are looking at. Your hands are resting on the edges of the foot, with the thumbs on the sole. You are starting just before the anklebone, where the foot bends. Walk all the fingers in slowly, feeling in between each bone. (See Figure 14.1.) The fingers look and act as though they are playing an accordion.

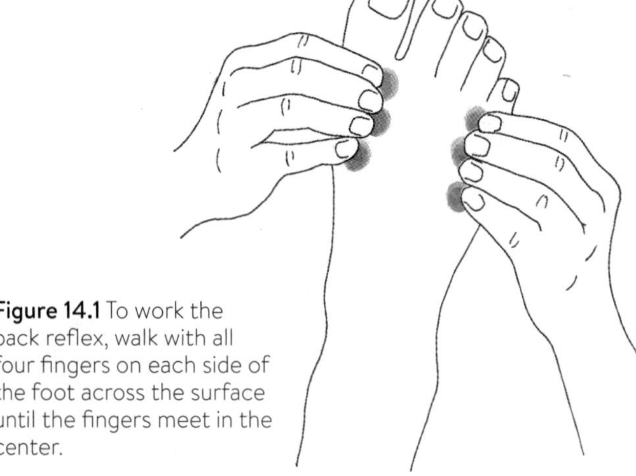

Figure 14.1 To work the back reflex, walk with all four fingers on each side of the foot across the surface until the fingers meet in the center.

Continue to finger walk in toward the center until the fingers meet. Move up slightly, bring the fingers back to the edge, and walk in again. Each time your fingers meet at the center, shift up slightly, bring the fingers back to the edge of the foot, and walk in again. Follow this procedure up to the base of the toes.

At the base of the toes, turn all the fingers down toward the ankle. The palms of the hands are at the top of the foot. Finger walk down the foot; again, this is in between the toes, just from a different angle. Walk all the way to just before the ankle and then slide back.

The Muscles and Bones of the Back

The reflexology techniques employed to work the back reflexes are working on reflex areas that are representative of this region of the body. As the circulation improves throughout the body, often the muscles in the back area begin to relax. When someone has a horrific backache and cannot stand to be touched, reflexology is a great tool.

Solar Plexus

You have reflexed a number of areas on the foot, and pressing into the solar plexus lets you bring a conclusion to this segment of the treatment. Working the solar plexus reflex is a reminder to the receiver and to the giver to breathe and flow with the movement of the work. Press your right thumb into the solar plexus reflex, pull the toes down toward the thumb; ask the receiver to take a slow, deep breath, and hold. Keep pressing as you instruct the receiver to release the breath slowly. Gently remove the thumb and let the toes relax as well.

Butterfly and Flutter

As you prepare to move on to the next section, it's time to use a transitional move. Using both hands, walk the thumbs and fingers together toward the center of the foot, working up and then down the foot. All the digits are involved in a butterfly movement. If you find this too confusing, work the top surface and then the bottom surface.

Once the butterfly has been employed, use the tips of the fingers to make fluttery movements on the top surface of the foot. Move from the ankle area to the toes, repeating this technique.

You have worked the upper portion of the foot, reflexing points connecting to the body from the waist up. The receiver is relaxed, and you are ready to move on.

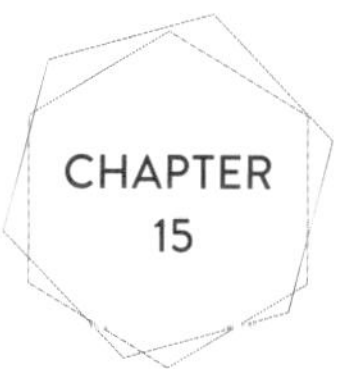

CHAPTER 15

Recharging the Digestive System

Take care of your body. It's the only place you have to live.
—JIM ROHN

The digestive system is a two-part mechanism. First, we eat food and assimilate the nutrients. Then we need to eliminate the waste. It sounds simple, but there is an incredible amount of work involved in this entire process—not to mention a lot of organs. Too much stress can disrupt the process, creating problems for the body. In this chapter, you'll learn how to recharge the digestive system so that the receiver can relax and let the digestion process function easily and naturally. You'll identify the corresponding zones of the foot that reflect everything from the colon to the small intestines to the bladder. And you'll discover how to apply the techniques you already know to this section of the foot.

From the Waistline to the Sciatic Line

The waistline is the guideline in the center of the arch. The sciatic line is found in the top section of the heel bone. Look at the bottom of the foot; you are still on the right foot. The instep is shaped as an arch, with the waistline running through the center.

Trace the heel bone, which begins at the end of the arch and ends at the back of the foot. The heel is covered with protective connective tissue and muscle. This covering gives the heel its puffy, fatty feeling as you push on the bone. The sciatic line runs about a finger joint down from the beginning of the heel. Another way to picture the sciatic line is to draw an imaginary line from the bony protrusion of the anklebone down to the heel and across to the other side.

You now have two lines marking the section you will be working on. The waistline is one line and the sciatic line is another. Draw an imaginary line along the inside edge from waistline to the sciatic line and draw another on the outside edge. Again you have made a long rectangular box, which will contain many reflexes.

Discovering Landmarks

In anatomy there are many surface landmarks, and a number of them are found on the feet. The bony bump at the end of the fifth metatarsal bone is such a landmark. Remember, this is the bone that helps to determine one edge of the waistline guideline. When you put your thumb across the bottom of the foot from this bony protuberance, you divide the arch, creating the waistline.

Some of the landmarks deal with muscles—the placement of muscles in relationship to their function. Some are the bony points that muscles attach to. Other landmarks deal with blood supply, marking the area of primary flow. Still other landmarks represent nerve placement. Some landmarks denote direction or movement. There are many such landmarks on the feet and ankles.

Locating the Landmarks

Some of the landmarks are on the top and sides of the foot:

- The medial malleolus is the high spot on the inside of the anklebone.
- The lateral malleolus is the high spot on the outside of the anklebone.
- The great saphenous vein is on top of the foot.

- The saphenous nerve is on top of the foot.
- The extensor digitorum brevis are muscles on top of the foot.
- The dorsalis pedis artery is on the top of the foot.
- The dorsal venous arch is on top of the foot.

Some of the landmarks are on the bottom of the foot. These are bony protuberances with odd shapes for connective tissue attachment:

- Sesamoid bones, under the head of the first metatarsal
- Base of the first metatarsal
- Head of the fifth metatarsal
- Tuberosity of the navicular
- Tuberosity of the fifth metatarsal
- Tuberosity of the calcaneus

Some of the landmarks are on the back of the foot:

- The peroneus longus and brevis are muscles and tendons from the leg.
- The small saphenous vein is on the back of the ankle.
- The sural nerve comes in around the back of the ankle.
- The tendo calcaneus is connected to the heel.
- The flexor hallucis longus is a muscle to the great toe.
- The posterior tibial artery is on the back of the ankle.
- The posterior tibial nerve is on the back of the ankle.

These landmarks might be used to explain a direction for a reflex technique. At times, these landmarks remind you of the movement the foot can make at these areas. These landmarks may denote the placement of a reflex point. For example, the area of a sciatic reflex point is connected to the actual nerve placement. Often you will notice this link between reflexes and landmarks.

• • • Reflex Points • • •

Two landmarks, the medial and lateral malleolus, form the bony area called the ankle. The true anklebone actually sits in between these bony ends of the lower leg. It is known as the talus. The ankle area consists of the seven tarsal bones plus the two malleoli.

The Ileocecal/Appendix Reflex

Look at the feet for a moment, placing them together with the soles facing you. Let yourself imagine the entire body superimposed over the feet. Take a moment to picture the head at the toes and slowly move down, seeing the different parts of the body as your eyes travel down the feet.

Stop just below the waistline. Imagine the waistline going right across the two feet. Move down from the waistline and feel along the outside edge of the foot. Look at the tuberosity of the fifth metatarsal; this is the bump at the bottom outside edge of the long bone that follows after the little toe on both feet. This bony landmark will guide you to find certain points in this next segment. Cover the left foot, as you will deal with the right foot first.

Hooking the Reflex

Hold the right foot with the right hand; the left hand gently cups the foot, with the thumb resting on the sole surface. Find the bony protuberance of the fifth metatarsal. Place the left thumb at this tuberosity and turn the thumb slightly down and in, preparing to thumb walk. Only the first digit of the thumb is actually in use at this moment. The rounded beginning surface of the heel is touching the edge of this thumb. This section of the thumb is in between the outside edge of the foot and the rounded edge of the heel on the bottom of the foot. The tip of the thumb is dropping into the reflex for the ileocecal valve.

Once you have pinpointed this reflex, which represents the ileocecal valve and the appendix, push in and gently rotate. Continue to rotate as the thumb moves in deeper, then gently push and hold on the point. The fingers of your working hand are being used as levers, supporting the back of the foot as the thumb pushes in. The right hand continues as the holding hand.

With the thumb pushed in and holding, pull back a bit toward the edge of the foot in the hooking technique. Push in a little more if possible while hooking. (See Figure 15.1.) This reflex is important as it represents the beginning of the large intestine. You work the large and small intestines together in much of this segment, as these areas of the body overlap.

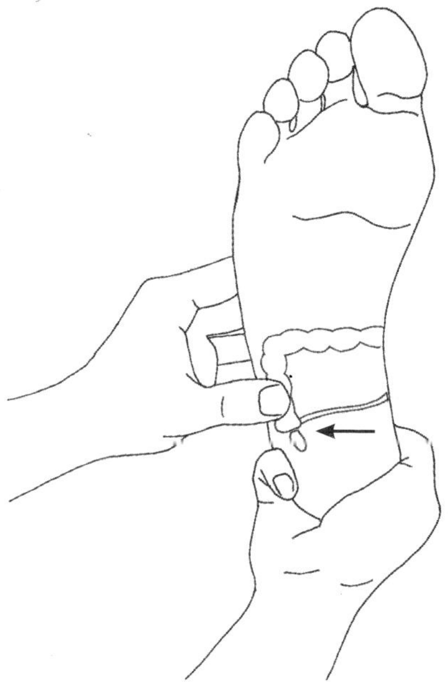

Figure 15.1 Pinpoint the ileocecal reflex with the hook in and back up technique.

The Gatekeeper

This reflex may be reflexed a number of times, as it represents a structure that is a gatekeeper. Throughout the body there are various small structures that hold positions of great functional importance. In the digestive system alone there are five such structures. In this system these are valves that allow materials to pass along the roadway of digestion. Sphincters are generally tight rings of muscle that permit passage in only one direction.

The Ascending Colon Reflex

The left thumb is hooked into the ileocecal valve reflex in a horizontal position. Turn the thumb up toward the waistline and begin to thumb walk up toward the waistline guideline. Take small, slow bites as the thumb walks up, creating a line close to the edge of the foot. The thumb is on the bottom surface but near the outside edge. This is the ascending colon reflex.

The right foot holds the reflexes for the ascending colon and half of the transverse colon. Bring the thumb back to the ileocecal reflex and thumb walk up the edge again. Feel how the foot responds. The reflex for the ascending colon is along the edge of the plantar surface and may feel tough to the touch at first, as this area is used for balance. The more the reflex is worked, the softer the skin will feel. The more relaxed the receiver, the easier it is to work the reflex.

The Hepatic Flexure and Transverse Colon Reflexes

The reflex for the colon is broken up into parts. Start at the outside edge of the waistline as you begin to thumb walk across this line to the inside edge. Let the thumb work at the outside edge first, with rotation and circling on the area. This is the hepatic flexure reflex. Thumb walk on the point in three directions, after the rotation and circling is completed. The thumb will take one or two tiny bites up, across, and down on the area of the flexure reflex.

Thumb walk across the bottom of the foot, along the waistline guide. This is the transverse colon reflex. At the inside edge of the foot, turn the thumb down, just a bit. The area where the thumb has stopped will pop out slightly. Use the right thumb to circle gently on the part of the skin that has pushed out. This is the top of the bladder reflex. You will be working on the entire reflex later. The transverse colon reflex is on both feet, as the piece of the colon it represents moves across the body near the stomach and the spleen.

Working All the Right Angles

From the ileocecal valve reflex, up the ascending colon reflex, across the transverse colon reflex, and all the secondary reflexes, this walk is reflecting half of the large intestine. At the same time, the small intestine in the body is intertwined with its larger counterpart, allowing for the overlapping of reflexes. Whew, what a mouthful, or should we say bellyful!

This first walk-through has created a different shape than those you have previously drawn. Look at the foot and imagine a line from the ileocecal reflex up and across the transverse colon reflex. This line would look like a right angle. Keep this image in mind as you move forward in this complex area.

The Second and Third Angles

Bring the left thumb back to the ileocecal valve reflex; rotate on the point and hold. Walk the thumb in two tiny steps away from the ileocecal reflex, toward the inside edge of the foot, and then turn and thumb walk up to the waistline. Just below the waistline guide, turn the thumb, moving toward the inside edge of the foot. Thumb walk across, making a line to the medial edge. This is now the second right angle, stacked under the first.

Bring the thumb back to the ileocecal valve point to begin a new right angle. Walk the thumb in from the valve reflex to just past where the last segment began. Thumb walk up toward the waistline again, stopping right below the line that was created by the last walk-through. Turn and work toward the center of the foot again. A third right angle has been created, tucked just inside the previous one.

Right-Angle Finale

Depending upon the size of the foot, the next right angle may be the last. Starting at the ileocecal valve reflex, thumb walk across the other lines to begin a new section. Turn and thumb walk up, turning again just below the last line across. Thumb walk to the inside edge of the foot, completing the final right angle. Notice that each time the pattern becomes smaller, as the area involved is less.

These stacked right angles have worked the areas of the large and small intestines as reflected on the right foot.

Create a Fan with Thumb Walking

You have worked the section relating to the small and large intestine on the right side of the body as you built the series of stacked right angles. Now you will work the area again, as this represents part of the system that rids the body of waste, supporting homeostasis. Also, since this area of the foot is often neglected, reflexology improves its tone, restoring much of the vibrancy to the skin and muscles.

Start with the left thumb rotating on the ileocecal reflex, move in, and hook. Gently turn the thumb and walk up the ascending colon reflex. Bring the thumb back to the valve reflex, hold on the point, and then thumb walk up again, next to the ascending colon reflex, to the waistline. Return the left thumb to the ileocecal reflex and hold; visualize the next line up, and thumb walk it.

Imagine a dancer holding a closed fan. The dance begins with the fan closed. With each twirl around the floor the dancer opens the fan a little more. The base of the fan is constant as the patterns on the pieces of the fan tell a story with each opening.

• • • Reflex Points • • •

The fan has effectively worked the section of the foot between the waistline and the sciatic guidelines. The steady, gentle thumb walking has allowed this part of the foot to feel relaxed and renewed.

The reflex for the ileocecal valve is the base of the fan and each line up and out is a strut of the fan. Each time the line ends, at the waistline, return to the ileocecal reflex and thumb walk another line out, opening the fan wider each time. Every thumb walk out will bring the thumb farther along the waistline, closer to the inner edge of the foot. Eventually the line will no longer go to the waistline but out to the inside edge of the foot. Ultimately the last line of the fan will end with the thumb walking away from the ileocecal reflex along the sciatic line to the inner side of the foot.

The Small Intestine Reflex Box

You have built a stack of right angles and created and opened a fan, techniques that relate to both the large and small intestines. The outside areas of the right angles dealt with the large intestine, as did the fan before it opened. You also have a reflex specific to the small intestines.

Look at the right foot and imagine the ileocecal valve reflex. Imagine, too, the ascending and transverse colon reflexes. There is an empty, open boxlike space to the inside and under these reflexes. Now imagine the box filled with squiggly lines, running in from the medial edge of the foot. Switch hands; you will be using your right thumb now.

Start thumb walking just under the waistline from the inside edge of the foot. Walk in to the hepatic reflex. Bring the thumb back to the edge and down a bit, and thumb walk back in again to the ascending colon reflex. Keep bringing the thumb back to the inside edge, a little lower every time. Continue to thumb walk, making imaginary lines and filling this box to the sciatic line.

Once the sciatic line has been thumb walked, fill the box in from the bottom up. This reflex for the small intestine can be worked from the top to the bottom, from the bottom to the top, and diagonally too. Imagine the 200-odd inches of the small intestine. Think, too, of all the work the small intestine does.

Kidney and Bladder Reflexes

On the bottoms of both feet there are reflexes for the kidneys, ureters, and bladder. The reflex for the kidney on the right foot is slightly lower than on the left. In the body, the kidneys are attached to the back wall of the abdomen, sitting just about at the waistline.

• • • Reflex Points • • •

People are many sizes and shapes, so each body has slightly different areas for placement of its internal organs. A tall, slimly built person may have a greater portion of the kidneys below the waist, whereas in a short, tiny person, the kidneys may sit above the waist. The body is the same yet individually unique.

The Kidney Reflex

You will work on the right foot, as the technique is the same on both feet. Refresh your memory on the location of the adrenal reflex. Hold the foot with the right hand and thumb walk toward the adrenal reflex with the left thumb. Work on the waistline as you thumb walk toward the centerline. Stop at the adrenal reflex, letting the thumb sit on the reflex and the waistline.

Imagine the little kidney bean shape superimposed on the foot, some above and some below the waistline. Keep cupping the foot at the heel with the right hand. Free the fingers of the left hand, as they are going to move over and around the foot. Keeping the left thumb on the reflex, swing the fingers over the top of the foot.

The fingers have moved from the dorsal surface, over the toes, to gently grasp the inner side of the foot, from the plantar side. You are now looking at the top of the palm of the left hand. The fingers are wrapped around the toes, resting on the dorsal surface, so you cannot see them. The left thumb is flat on the sole, resting completely on the foot. The kidney reflex is this entire area under the thumb, above and below the waistline. (See Figure 15.2.) Gently rotate the thumb in, press, and hold. Do not apply excess pressure, as this is a sensitive area.

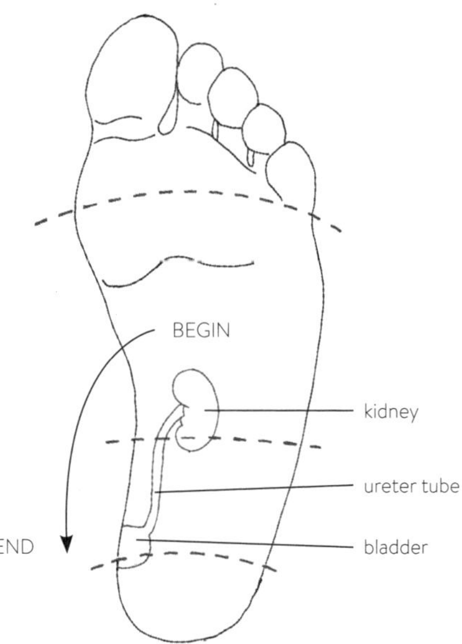

Figure 15.2 Thumb walk across the waistline into the kidney reflex, and rotate on the point before thumb walking down to the bladder reflex.

The Bladder Reflex

Look at the foot for a moment, visualizing the path the next reflex will take. From the kidney reflex, thumb walk down diagonally to the lower inner edge of the foot, by the sciatic line. Watch as the area here begins to pop out; this will tell you that you're working the reflex correctly! When the thumb reaches the edge of the foot, there is a slight bulge of the fatty tissue area; this is the bladder reflex. Using your right thumb, gently circle and thumb walk on this region. Thumb walk gently in all directions on this reflex, then softly flutter off.

The Heel in Transition

You have worked the reflexes of digestion, absorption, and elimination on the right foot. You will now begin to work on the finishing touches that will complete the main portion of the session on the right foot. Either hand can be used as the working hand, with the other hand holding the foot for support and leverage. First you want to work the sciatic line, as this is one of the areas of reflection for the sciatic nerve.

• • • Reflex Points • • •

At times the hands may feel tired as the muscles are strengthening. If a working hand is tired, transitions are a great time to give the hand a rest.

Heel Press

Form the working hand into a fist, then press into the heel as though kneading dough. Press over the entire heel area, back and forth and up and down. This area may be tough and have hardened skin. As you press on the heel, you can feel the toughness beginning to relax, responding to the work. Continue to press on the heel until the response is felt on the entire area.

Thumb Walk the Sciatic Line

The sciatic line has been relaxed with the heel press, ready for a deeper technique. Using either the right or left thumb, walk across the line, starting from either edge. Thumb walk slowly, feeling the area respond. When the thumb reaches the end of the imaginary line, either switch hands and walk back or bring the thumb back to the beginning edge and walk across again.

Reflexologists often thumb walk and heel press, using both techniques interchangeably here. Allow yourself to see what works for you.

Moving On

As you complete this section, flutter off in transition. Let the hands rest for a moment on the entire foot, cupping both sides. With soft movements, allow your hands to gently stroke or flutter off, giving the signal to rest. In a complete session, you would continue on with this foot. However, this is a learning session, so cover the right foot and get ready to go over to the left foot.

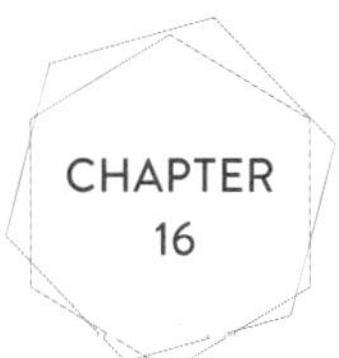

CHAPTER 16

Digestion and the Left Foot

We have much to learn by studying nature and taking the time to tease out its secrets.

—*DAVID SUZUKI*

Any modality worth studyinq has sections of ease and areas of complexity. However, reflexology becomes less demanding with practice. Let's go ahead and move to the left foot, and you can practice more along the way. In this chapter, you'll discover the reflexes of the digestive system as they're reflected in the left foot. You'll learn more landmarks and create more fans and right angles (as you did in the previous chapter), and you'll use the same basic techniques as before, such as thumb walking and knuckle pressing. The main challenge is finding the correct place on the foot to work, and don't be surprised if this quickly becomes second nature to you.

The Left Foot

You have steadily been working on the right foot, with the exception of the warm-up routine and the examination of the spleen reflex. Now it is time to deal with the left foot as you approach the left side of the body. Energetically, the left side of the body represents the sunny side of the slope. The concept of yin and yang can be equated with the concept of homeostasis. One deals with energetic balance and the other deals with physical balance. The combination of the two will create the perfect setting for spiritual balance. A smooth flow of chi along the energy channels in the body creates good health. To achieve this flow we must operate in harmony.

Much of the flow of movement in the body is from right to left. The digestive system moves the waste out from right to left, and the left foot holds the outward flow reflexes of this system. The lungs oxygenate the blood as it flows from the right side into the left.

Placement of Organs

The left side of the body holds the larger portion of the heart. This side also has a greater piece of the stomach. The pancreas in some people has a bit more on the left side. One half of the transverse colon is on the left side of the body. The descending colon and the sigmoid colon are found on the left side as well. The rectum is in the center of the body; however, the reflex is generally located on the left foot, in line with the sigmoid colon.

The Gastrointestinal Tract

This section of the reflexology session deals with the lower part of the gastrointestinal tract. The gastrointestinal tract (GI tract) has been discussed briefly during the discussion of the digestive system. Working these reflexes will continue to support the digestive system.

• • • Reflex Points • • •

The left foot mirrors the right foot, with the same structures in the same places. All the bones are the same, as are the entire accessory structures connected with the feet.

Creating the Outside Box

Look at the foot and picture the waistline running across the center. Find the tuberosity of the fifth metatarsal, that bony bump at the outside edge, and place your thumb in from here across the center of the foot. There is the waistline guide for this foot. Look at the heel and feel that area of the foot. Grasp the heel, become familiar with the feel on all sides. For reference, feel your way around your own heel.

Use all your fingers and walk all over the heel. Extend the foot away and feel the tautness. Flex the foot in and notice how the top end of the heel relaxes somewhat. The end of the heel is at the back of the foot; feel from the back along the bottom surface to the beginning of this structure.

Let your fingers move down the heel on the plantar side, toward the back just a bit, perhaps a joint length. Here the heel is puffy and tight, yet the area does respond. This is the sciatic line region. Begin at the outside edge of the foot and thumb walk across the heel, making an imaginary line. Bring the thumb back and walk again.

Now begin to practice on a receiver. The left hand is holding the foot and the right hand is walking. Switch hands and let the left thumb walk along the sciatic line from the inside of the foot. Bring the thumb back to the inside edge and walk along the line again. Always be aware of the response from the foot, checking to feel if the foot is relaxing.

Thumb Walk the Transverse Reflex

Hold the left foot with the right hand as you use the left thumb to walk along the waistline. The fingers of the left hand may be tucked in a loose fist or rest on the top surface of the foot, whichever works for you. Begin at the inside edge of the waistline and, using small, slow bites, thumb walk across the transverse colon reflex.

Continue to thumb walk along this line, tilting up a bit toward the spleen reflex. As the left thumb reaches the outside edge, you will feel a slight indentation. Switch hands now; the right thumb will take over. Using the right thumb, move into the area that is slightly up from the waistline in the outside corner. This is where the indentation is located.

This slight depression represents the splenic flexure in the colon. A flexure is an area of the colon that bends, creating a pocket or reservoir where waste may become stuck. This side of the body has two such flexures.

Using the right thumb, hook into this reflex. Remember to rotate on the spot, press, and hold, feeling how deeply in the foot it's allowing you to go. Then hook in and pull back, as though the reflex was the fish and the thumb the fishhook.

Thumb Walk Down the Descending Colon Reflex

The descending colon reflex moves from the splenic flexure down the outside edge of the foot, past the bony tuberosity of the fifth metatarsal. The reflex continues to the sciatic line where the descending colon reflex ends.

With the right thumb already in position, turn slightly and thumb walk down the descending colon reflex. This may seem awkward at first since you are using the tip and the inside edge of the thumb. The inside edge here means the edge farthest away from the index finger.

• • • Reflex Points • • •

The medial side of the thumb and great toe are actually the sides that touch each other. This means that what looks like the outside edge is really the inside edge. Let your arms hang down at the sides of your body. The inside edge of the thumbs, the medial edge, is the edge closest to the body.

Take a look at what has happened so far. You have walked across the transverse colon reflex, which turns up a bit just under the spleen reflex. Under the spleen reflex is the reflex for the splenic flexure; here the techniques used were rotation, press, hook, and hold on the point. From the splenic flexure reflex, you turned the thumb to face downward and used the thumb-walking technique, this time down the descending colon, ending at the sciatic guideline.

The Bony Landmark

The fifth metatarsal on the left foot is used as a guide along much of the process on this foot. The descending colon reflex runs to the end of this bone, meeting the tuberosity of this fifth long bone. Just past this bony landmark there is a depression in the bottom surface of the foot. The small space, which feels like a tiny gap, is a reflex.

Trace your finger down the fifth metatarsal bone. Press in and feel the bone, letting your finger come to the end, and feel the bumpy protrusion. Feel past the tuberosity and discover the depression just in and under that bone. The fifth metatarsal is in front of the cuboid bone. The cuboid bone is also behind the fourth metatarsal. The muscles and tendons that are connected to the cuboid and these metatarsals are interwoven like a wicker chair. The space that represents a reflex is part of this area. The crisscrossing of the muscles, tendons, and ligaments has left a slight depression that you can feel. The reflex is the sigmoid colon flexure. This small area reflects the final turn in the colon.

Thumb walk across the transverse colon with the left thumb. Switch to the right thumb and hook into the splenic flexure. Thumb walk down the descending colon. Allow the right thumb to walk into the slight depression under the bony landmark. With the right thumb, rotate on this point, press, and hold. Use the thumb to hook in and pull back, hooking into this reflex. (See Figure 16.1.)

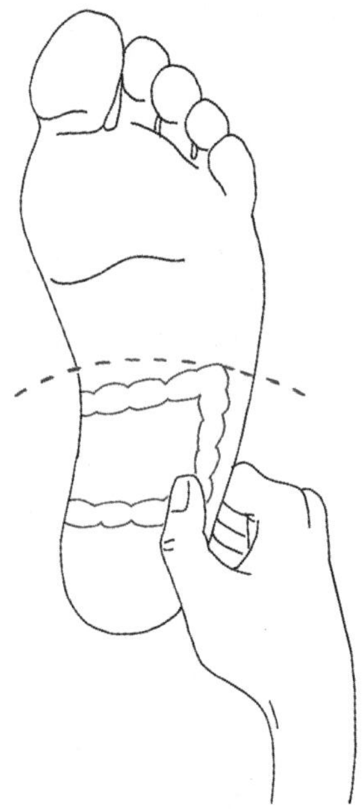

Figure 16.1 Using the right thumb, hook in and rotate on the sigmoid reflex.

Rotate on the Rectal Reflex

Thumb walk across the left foot, from the last flexure reflex, over the fleshy top part of the heel, just above the sciatic line, to the inside edge. Take small steps, using a slow, even motion with the thumb-walking technique. Feel the foot responding to the pressure. Walk completely across the foot, over the edge, into another slight depression. This small space is just past the ridge on the inside of the foot, about at the tuberosity of the navicular.

This depression is the rectal reflex. The right thumb walks into the space first, presses in, and holds. The left thumb will move into the gap and take over. Feel how the thumb dips in a bit, as this area is flexible. Use caution here; do not press too hard, as this reflex point is often sensitive. Rotate on the reflex and hold.

The Box Is Complete

Look at the bottom of the foot where you have just worked. In essence you have created another box, an odd-shaped rectangular box. Using the two imaginary guidelines along with the reflexes, you can imagine this irregular box shape:

- Waistline guideline
- Transverse colon reflex
- Splenic flexure reflex
- Descending colon reflex
- Sigmoid flexure reflex
- Sigmoid colon reflex
- Rectal reflex
- Sciatic guideline

This represents the first complete walk-through of the left segment reflecting the large intestine. Of course the small intestines are also represented, which will receive attention in the next segment.

More Right Angles

Ready to have some fun? With this technique you'll alternate using both thumbs. Hold the foot with the right hand, bring the left thumb to the waistline, and close the left hand in a loose fist or let the fingers rest lightly on the top of the foot. Thumb walk across the center of the foot, along the transverse colon reflex.

At the splenic flexure reflex, switch hands. The left hand holds the foot steady while the right hand works. Using the right thumb, with the fingers closed in a loose fist, turn and thumb walk down the descending colon reflex. Leave the right hand there for the moment holding the foot, and return to the left thumb.

Begin with the left thumb just a bit under the transverse reflex at the inner edge of the foot, and walk to the outside edge again, across the foot. Stop just before the splenic flexure reflex. Let the left hand hold there, as you will use the right thumb now.

Using the right thumb to do the work, walk down the foot, alongside and just in from the descending reflex to the sciatic line. Again leave the right hand there, returning to use the left. Bring the left thumb down slightly, and, starting at the inner edge, thumb walk across, stopping at the line just inside the descending reflex. Using the right thumb, walk down from this point to the sciatic line. Look at what has happened. You have created a group of stacked right angles again, one inside the other. Generally, three to four little stools are what you can construct on the bottom of the foot.

Draw Another Fan

With the last sequence you worked the reflexes for the large and small intestines, but you aren't finished yet! The receiver might be reporting grumbles and gurgles emanating from the belly and intestinal regions. You may even hear these sounds. This is an affirmation that you are doing a great job, working to relax the recipient.

The Fan's Base

Begin by using the right thumb and walk down the descending colon reflex, stopping at the sigmoid flexure reflex. At this juncture, let the thumb slip into the slight depression, rotate to move in deeply, hold while pressing, and hook this reflex. The left hand is holding the foot. The right thumb is doing the reflexing; the right fingers are either coiled in a loose fist or resting on the top surface of the foot. Hold on this point for a moment, really pinpointing the reflex. You are going to build another fan; however, this fan will be slightly different than the one on the right foot.

Fanning Out

Look at the area you are working on. Imagine a line drawn from the sigmoid flexure reflex diagonally across the foot up to the inner waistline. The line will come across the inner arch, reaching up to find the beginning of the transverse colon. This will be the first swipe of the fan—when the dancer is holding the fan closed, waiting to proceed.

Return your gaze to the sigmoid flexure reflex and again imagine a line, this time going across just under the first line. Here the fan would begin to open. If you were drawing this, you would continue to return to the flexure reflex and keep drawing lines out until eventually the fan would be completely open, with the open end terminating on the length of the sigmoid colon reflex along the sciatic line.

• • • Reflex Points • • •

Imagining the sequence before you actually perform the work is always a good practice. Feeling the area of the foot, drawing on paper, or drawing on the foot makes it a natural progression from our imagination. It's much easier to perform if you give yourself the image to work with.

Thumb walk the reflex now. Begin at the sigmoid flexure reflex with the right thumb, using the left hand as the holding hand. The left hand will be supporting the foot either by holding the toes or with the hand placed firmly across the center dorsal surface. Press in and rotate on the flexure reflex. Then slowly thumb walk diagonally across the instep toward the beginning of the transverse colon.

Return to the flexure reflex and repeat this process, following just inside the diagonal line as the thumb moves across the foot. Each time, the thumb returns to the flexure and works diagonally across, reaching the inner edge of the foot as the lines of the fan open. The last line begins with the sigmoid flexure reflex and the thumb walks straight across the sigmoid colon reflex.

A Box for the Small Intestine Reflex

The small intestine reflex is the same on both sides of the body. Recognizing these reflexes lets you put a finishing touch on the digestive segment.

Building the Box

You have built an oddly shaped box that reflects the large intestine. Within that box is an open area that serves as the small intestine reflex. Starting at the inside edge of the foot, from just below the waistline, walk in slowly toward the outside edge of the foot. You are using your left thumb, taking small, deep bites across the foot. When you reach the descending colon reflex, bring the thumb back immediately to the inside edge.

Again thumb walk in, this time starting slightly lower, just under the line you just created. Continue to walk in with the left thumb, moving down each time until eventually you stop just above the sigmoid colon reflex. Generally, you can make three or four lines before you reach the sigmoid reflex. Switch hands, and with the right thumb walk back up and across the area you just worked.

You are creating a pattern across the foot on the small intestine reflex, like the lattice topping of a pie. Either or both thumbs may move around in this reflex, until you feel a softening of the skin. This softening is a signal that the foot has relaxed in this area.

Revisiting the Kidney and Bladder

The body has two kidneys that both empty into the bladder. To access this reflex on the left foot is fairly straightforward. Begin at the transverse colon reflex, and, using the left thumb, thumb walk in to the tendon line near the center of the foot. The kidney reflex sits on, above, and below this line, which is located directly under the solar plexus reflex. The adrenal reflex sits on top of the kidney reflex, which helps in finding the point.

Once the thumb is on the reflex, switch hands, since you will be thumb walking back toward the inside of the foot. Let the left hand hold the foot now, while the right thumb settles on the reflex. Turn the right thumb; the entire thumb will rest on the reflex, facing down toward the heel. Bring the fingers across the top of the toes and gently grasp the foot. The fingers will hold around the toes as the top of the hand rests on the bottom of the foot.

Turn the thumb slightly in toward the lower inner edge of the foot. Thumb walk down from the kidney reflex, along the ureter reflex, until the thumb reaches the edge of the foot. Walk just a bit farther, and the thumb will push out the bladder reflex. Use the left thumb now to gently circle on the reflex. This is a very soothing technique, allowing for deeper relaxation connected with calming touch.

Ahhh, Knuckle Press the Heel

To perform the knuckle press, use either hand as the working hand. Hold the foot steady and press the flat surface of the closed fist on the heel. Let the knuckles knead the heel, moving back and forth across the entire area. Feel the skin soften and the area become more giving.

Using the heel press is a terrific way to close this section of the treatment. The heel will always welcome and thank you for paying it extra attention. So many of us abuse our feet, particularly the heel area. Walking incorrectly, made worse by ill-fitting shoes, is one of the causes of heel pain. The heel generally supports 25 percent of your body weight.

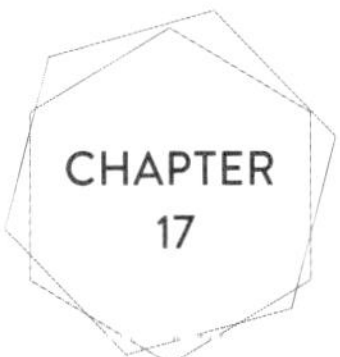

Reflexing the Reproductive System

The greatest miracle on Earth is the human body.
It is stronger and wiser than you probably realize.
And improving its ability to heal is within your control.
—*DR. FABRIZIO MANCINI*

The reproductive system is an incredible piece of symmetry. The areas reflected on the feet for this system are the same on both the right and the left foot. Both sexes are represented on the feet in the same or a similar way, as the structures and organs of the reproductive system are placed in very similar locations in the body. In this chapter, you'll put to use all of the techniques and concepts covered in previous chapters and find out how to use them to reflex the reproductive system. Ready for more thumb walking and shape making? Let's get started!

Bony Landmarks—the Ankles

The bony landmarks that represent the ankles are actually the ends of the two lower leg bones, the tibia and the fibula. The bony protrusions are called the medial and lateral malleolus. The medial malleolus is the end of the tibia, which sits on the inside of the foot. The lateral malleolus is the end of the fibula, which sits on the outside of the foot.

The ankle actually consists of all the tarsal bones. The talus is considered the real anklebone and is the initial weight-bearing bone during the action of walking.

Joints

Another area of importance in dealing with the ankle is the joint involved with the movement of this area. A joint is a point of contact between bones. The ankle joint is also known as the talocrural joint. It is between the end of the malleoli and the talus. This joint is classified structurally as a hinge joint. Part of the classification stipulates that the surface of one bone fits into the surface of another bone, which does happen in the ankles. The movement of the joint is like a door on a hinge; in anatomy this movement is generally flexion and extension. When you flex a joint it is as though you pull the door in, and when you extend, you open the door.

Special Movements

The synovial joints have a subgroup known as special movements. These movements are part of the biomechanics of the feet. Every time you walk you perform these special movements. Six of these special movements deal specifically with the feet and hands:

1. Inversion moves the soles inward, so they face each other.
2. Eversion moves the soles away, so they face away from each other.
3. Dorsiflexion bends the foot up.
4. Plantar flexion bends the foot down.
5. Abduction moves the foot away from the center of the body.
6. Adduction moves the foot toward the center of the body.

Although not special movements, there are two others that are key to some of these movements: The first is called supination, which is a three-point movement of inversion, plantar flexion, and adduction. The second is called pronation, which is a three-point movement of eversion, dorsiflexion, and abduction.

Reflexes on the Inside Arch

Hold the right foot with the left hand and knuckle press the heel. Press with a kneading movement; don't forget to move your body. Let the press relax the heel. Move up and down the plantar surface of this foot, using a gentle pressure and allowing the knuckles to relax the entire foot. Turn the foot out slightly and move your body so that you are looking at the inside edge of the foot, without twisting your neck and back. The reflexes found on the inside of the foot, in the lower arch and heel region, represent the reproductive system.

Thumb Walking a Triangle

Look at the inside of the foot and use the bony malleolus as a guide. Place a finger from the very edge of the heel up to just under the outside edge of the ankle. With the other hand, place a finger from the inside edge of the malleolus back toward the upper arch. Let the thumbs join each other along the inside edge of the foot. The shape between these fingers is a triangle.

Working the Reproductive Reflexes

Within this triangle are most of the reproductive reflexes. Some of these reflexes you will pinpoint; others you will include in the thumb-walking technique. Look at the shape once more and remove the fingers, preparing to thumb walk. Begin with the right thumb, and thumb walk up from the back of the heel to the outside of the malleolus. Keep moving the thumb in a bit and walk up so that the line continues to come from the inside edge of the foot up to the malleolus. Eventually using the right thumb becomes awkward, which is a sign to switch hands.

The left thumb walks the imaginary line that begins along the edge of the foot at the waistline. Thumb walk along this line to just under the upper edge of the malleolus. Continue to bring the thumb back to the edge and walk with small, slow bites up to the ankle, but not on the bone. Soon the entire triangle is filled.

The line that runs from the edge of the heel to the waistline is next. Thumb walk between these two points. Return to the edge of the heel, move the thumb in a bit, and walk again. You are filling in the area from the heel to the bone on the side of the foot, the tuberosity of the navicular.

Reflexes of the Inner Triangle

There are many reflexes within this triangle. This area reflects the pelvic region of the body, including all structures found there. The area along the back edge of the heel has reflexes for the testes and lymph. Moving in a bit—just up from the inner edge but still close to the back—are two reflexes: one for the vaginal area and the other for the pelvic bones. The entire triangle is the reflex for the uterus.

The reflex for the rectum is a thumb joint in from the edge along the sciatic line. Thumb walking the triangle, from the heel, from the waistline, and filling in the whole area allows for complete coverage of all the reflexes. Other areas reflected here are the prostate gland and the urethra.

Press and Hold Behind the Ankle

Look at the inside of the foot for a moment. Focus on the medial malleolus. Feel around this bony area on your own foot. Become familiar with the dips and curves. Flex and extend the foot and move the foot in a circle while your fingers are palpating around this bony section. Place a fingertip in the space just behind the ankle. The finger slips into this small space easily. With the finger in this tiny section, turn the foot toward the finger and feel the finger press in.

You are using the body to work the reflex as the finger holds on the point. What you are feeling is the stimulation of the tibial nerve and the pulsing of the tibial artery. The tibial nerve is a main branch of the sciatic nerve. Surface veins are also in this area.

The sciatic line along the plantar surface of the foot is a reflex for the sciatic nerve. The reflex point just behind and below the malleolus is the sciatic point. Look at the receiver's foot and examine around the inner malleolus. When you are ready, thumb walk in from the edge of the foot, walking with small bites to just behind the inner ankle. Let your thumb fit into the small depression and hold there.

Pull the recipient's foot into the thumb. This is a sensitive region, so be easy and do not apply pressure; the foot will do the work.

Reflexes on the Outside of the Foot

Now you're ready to move on to the outside region of the feet—the right foot first, of course. There are many reflexes found here. Beginning with the heel area along the lower edge is a reflection found for the lymphatics. This runs around the entire region of the foot from the lower edge of the outside heel, up and across the navicular and talus on the top of the foot, and down to the lower edge of the inner heel. Connecting with this line is the reflex for the fallopian tubes as well as the vas deferens.

Becoming Familiar with the Reflexes

At the lower, back edge of the heel on the outside is a reflex for the ovaries; the finger can generally fit right into the groove. Behind and below the outside malleolus is the sciatic point again. Let your fingers explore around the malleolus on this side, slipping into the sciatic reflex, then walking all around the bony protrusion of the ankle. This outer anklebone is the reflex for the hip, the entire hip bone, and the hip joints. The pelvic bones are around this area too.

Slowly feel along the outer edge, moving up the foot. Your finger will find the bony bump of the tuberosity of the fifth metatarsal. Keep moving up. The next bony bump is the fifth metatarsal head. The first indentation, under the tuberosity, is a secondary access for the hip, knee, and leg. The next indentation is just before the fifth metatarsal head. This point is a secondary access for the shoulder, elbow, and arm.

Move back and look at the area below the malleolus. Place a finger from the back edge of the heel up to the ankle. With the other hand, place a finger from the waistline to the ankle. Using the thumbs, connect the triangle by placing the thumbs along the edge between the waistline and the end of the heel. This is the primary access to the hip, knee, and leg.

Technique for Lymph and Reproductive Reflexes

To work the lymphatic reflex, you will use both hands. Place the thumbs on the edge of the heel, one on each side of the foot. Fit the thumbs as far back as possible, touching the tuberosity of the heel on both sides. Begin thumb walking diagonally up and across the heel, still under the malleolus. Continue to walk up, past the malleolus to the center top of the foot. The thumbs will pass over many landmarks as they walk to the top. When the thumbs meet, gently press in and hold. Begin moving the thumbs backward, following the path just drawn. Let the thumbs rotate slightly as you bring them back to the heel. This also represents the fallopian tubes and vas deferens. These reflexes and the lymphatic reflex overlap.

Once this reflex has been walked, imagine a line from the bottom of the malleolus drawn straight down to the heel. Thumb walk halfway up this line, and the finger will fit into a small dent. This is another reflex for the ovaries and fallopian tubes. Rotate in gently, hold, and press on this reflex.

The sciatic nerve reflex is in the same spot as on the inside of the foot. Thumb walk in horizontally, from the edge of the heel to behind the bottom edge of the malleolus. Sure enough, there is that slight dip, waiting for your thumb. Press in and hold, pulling the foot toward the thumb.

Begin to thumb walk up the outside edge of the foot. As the thumb walks into the groove before the tuberosity, turn the thumb slightly and hold. Pull the foot in toward the thumb; the body will use the thumb to press the reflex. Continue on from here to the next tiny spot, just below the metatarsal head. Turn the thumb just a bit, holding there, and pull the foot into the thumb. Again, the body is applying the pressure to the reflex.

Another Triangle

This triangle is the one you previously traced on the outside of the heel. Let's review. Put your two thumbs and index fingers together in a pyramid or triangle shape. Move your body so you are at the side of the foot you are working on. Place these fingers over the side of the foot, with the peak coming to rest under or on that protruding anklebone.

This outer triangle represents reflexes for the hip, knee, and leg. The entire area is a reflex. Thumb walking this region will reflex the leg and feet, as well as the knee and hip. Using the right thumb, walk up the edge of the foot to the waistline. Bring the thumb back and over a bit and walk up again, this time moving into the imaginary triangle. Continue in this manner, filling the triangle from the heel edge.

When the thumb cannot go any farther, you have hit the underside of the malleolus. Start to walk down with the left thumb. The left thumb will walk from the waistline down, essentially repeating the technique from another direction.

Lastly, thumb walk with the right thumb from the side edge up toward the malleolus, filling in the area. Let the thumb walk all over this section, using gentle, small steps. This area may be painful, so always check the comfort level of the receiver.

Reflexing the Hips

The reflection of the hip, the hip joints, and the bones of the hip is found around the lateral malleolus. This is the big bumpy bone that sits on the outside of the ankle, the one most people call the anklebone. You have felt around this area before and know how sensitive it can be.

Start at the lower end of the bone and thumb walk toward the back, turning and thumb walking up behind the ankle. Generally, the thumb and hand begin to twist awkwardly at this point. Switch thumbs and walk down toward the front of the foot, around the malleolus. The turn of the thumbs will be a bit awkward; this is one time where the body doesn't completely adjust. Pay attention to any areas of puffiness or tautness, as you will need to thumb walk carefully in these regions.

PART 5
Putting It All Together

Tension is who you think you should be.
Relaxation is who you are.
—CHINESE PROVERB

CONGRATULATIONS! YOU'VE MADE it through basic training. In this part, the focus shifts to giving all of your new knowledge a framework so that you can go forward and practice appropriately. You'll learn how to apply the principles of reflexology in an intentional way. You'll also learn more about the use of reflexology with other modalities, such as Reiki. You'll be shown how to appropriately end a reflexology session and send your receiver out into the world in a calmer, less stressed frame of mind. And for the person who doesn't have a lot of time, you'll find out how to do a mini-session that can be nearly as restorative as a full session. Finally, you'll learn when it's not a good idea to do reflexology, such as when you or the receiver is contagious, and how to make modifications to a session, such as for a receiver who has an injury in the foot or leg, and other such considerations.

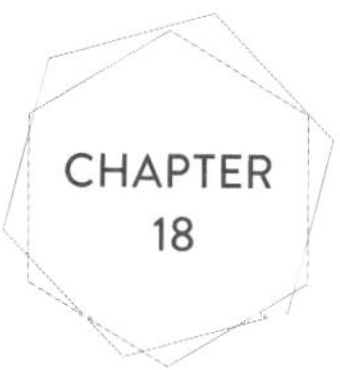

CHAPTER 18

Holistic Reflexology

It is health that is real wealth and not pieces of gold and silver.

—MAHATMA GANDHI

Reflexology is an energetic touch therapy that can help many people receive comfort and relief through healing touch. Each move within the techniques is applied with compassion. You reflex an area until you feel a response from the receiver. At times you may feel the reflex "give" as the skin beneath your finger or thumb relaxes. Sometimes there is a pulsation from the area of reflex. Or a reflex may "push" you away, a statement by the reflex that you should move on.

Feeling these responses comes with practice. The better you become with the art of reflexology, the easier it is for your hands to read the feet. As you gain knowledge and skill, you'll discover that reflexology can be enhanced with a deeper understanding of its connection to other modalities. With the help of this chapter, you can begin to grow in your knowledge of reflexology as a holistic practice.

A Reflexologist's Job

Do you ever have a day you just don't feel like going to work? The thought of going to your job just does not appeal to you. Imagine the value of always enjoying what you do, regardless of how you may be feeling personally.

A reflexologist's intention is to give the best session, to help in whatever way is appropriate, and to ensure the receiver is safe and secure. Reflexologists work in a systematic style, allowing for complete relaxation, in an environment that honors the receiver. They listen and respect what they are told, incorporating pertinent information. The person sitting in the reflexologist's chair trusts that the giver is providing what he or she needs.

Total Relaxation

The giver sets the stage for total relaxation for the receiver, allowing the receiver to release troubling or busy thoughts, permitting the muscles to let go of tension, and creating an environment dedicated to whole wellness.

Whole wellness is the concept of healing the whole person. The giver sets up an energy flow that creates a path allowing unrestricted use of the healing touch he is employing. Well-intentioned touch through reflexology promotes deep relaxation.

• • • Reflex Points • • •

Total relaxation allows the nervous system to activate a healing response. This response reaches out farther into the body, affecting the immune system. The process of homeostasis is a constant flow of balanced energy.

A Partnership of Wellness

Remember, you are not treating any specific condition, nor are you diagnosing any illness. What reflexology does, by viewing the receiver as a whole being, is to allow an atmosphere of wellness to become a real concept, incorporating both the giver and receiver in a partnership. This cooperative entity enables the receiver to take charge of his body, mind, and spirit, utilizing the tools the giver has introduced.

The value of wellness is a learned response. Many people do not realize the role they play in this concept. As you encourage the receivers to stand in their own place of power, this value becomes real.

• • • Reflex Points • • •

Psychoneuroimmunology is the study of how the mind and the body affect each other. Studies have proven that a positive state of mind creates a positive emotional environment that will support wellness. Disease is promoted by negative thoughts and emotions. Reflexology helps the receiver establish a harmonious attitude, generating the integration of body and mind wellness.

The Practice of Holistic Energy Medicine

Whole life healing is the practice of holistic energy medicine. What does that term mean? Holistic means whole. Energy means life. Medicine means to heal. This does not mean that reflexologists practice medicine. Far from it! Reflexologists and other energy workers assist the receiver in helping themselves by using the whole body concept. The only true healer is the body, mind, and spirit of the person being administered to. The integration of many modalities contributes to whole wellness.

All about Balance

The balance of all three elements—body, mind, and soul—is essential for true wellness. Being healthy is a many-faceted experience with many components. Physical health exists when all systems are functioning at their best for the individual, who is then full of zest and exuberance. A healthy environment is essential and includes the food you eat, the water you drink, and the air you breathe. Honoring your living space and those you live and work with is also part of whole health.

••• Reflex Points •••

Guided visualization is a tool you can use with reflexology or at any time to help you be healthy in body, mind, and soul. By using your imagination, along with specific thoughts, affirmations, pictures, sounds, and colors, you can create the space in which to reside during this journey through life.

Mental health is another part of the holistic picture. Living a satisfying life and feeling fulfilled by your experiences are necessary aspects of a balanced and mindful state of being. Emotional well-being is a key part of living your best life. A healthy spiritual self allows for unconditional connection and recognition of a Greater Source and a universal energy.

Create Your Own Reality

As you take charge of your wellness, begin to look at the concept of body, mind, and soul as tools to lead to good health. Try to understand how important it is to set a positive intention, allowing you to manifest a positive reality. You are what you eat, what you think, what you act, what you feel, and what you believe. Your well-being depends on the existence of internal harmony among these influences.

We all have heard that you can "create your own reality." As you become more involved with the homeostasis of self, you will recognize integration of the soul with the mind and the heart. If you decide you are going to have a good attitude, no matter what anyone else implies, you will have a good attitude. Creating a new reality that is happier, more content, and less frustrated will allow you to live in a better space, a space you have taken control of.

Reflexology and Other Modalities

Reflexology works well with other holistic healing techniques. Reiki, an energy-healing technique, and reflexology make a dynamic combination. Reiki techniques increase the effect of reflexology, supporting the balance and harmony that it promotes.

Acupressure, shiatsu, and acupuncture are all complemented with the addition of reflexology. Any massage session is more dynamic with reflexology included. A pedicure combined with reflexology keeps people coming back!

Reflexology in hospice is a compassionate and sensitive addition where touch is so important. Any inclusion of reflexology with contemporary treatment is a supportive addition. People recovering from surgeries, cancer treatments, or any other severe conditions report the use of reflexology as a welcome supplement.

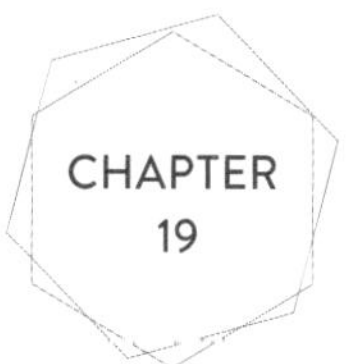

CHAPTER 19

Close Down, Cool Out

Without inner peace, outer peace is impossible.
—*GESHE KELSANG GYATSO*

The reflexology treatment is coming to a close, and you want to allow for a harmonious transition. In this chapter, you will discover how to effectively end a session on a positive, relaxed note. You will be shown how to close down and cool out, and how to use karate chops, tapping, and clapping to signal the end of a treatment. You'll also learn about a technique called the double solar plexus press. Further, this chapter examines why you shouldn't discount the importance of allowing the receiver a little peace and quiet at the end. Finally, this chapter discusses how to offer a mini-session—a shorter version of a full treatment—for those occasions when time is short.

Close Down

As you prepare to end the session, it is important to allow the receiver the time and space to become grounded and process what has just transpired. First, go back to each foot and work any reflex points that need more attention. These would be the reflexes that called to you during the session.

Perhaps an area was extra sensitive. Or a point resisted your fingers. Maybe another area was too pliable. The more you practice reflexology, the more aware and alert your fingers and your senses will become to the underlying tensions found in the feet.

Make a practice of gently walking the zones on each foot one last time (as shown in Figure 19.1), to ensure all reflex points have been properly worked. Walk your fingers down the tops of the feet and in between the metatarsal bones as a final walk-through. This is equivalent to a gentle cradling of the body, weaving together any loose ends.

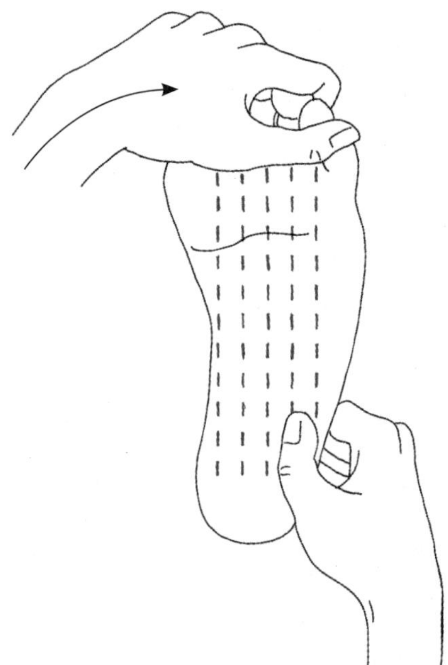

Figure 19.1 As you close down, walk the zones on each foot one last time.

Cool Out

After you have walked the zones one last time, place your hands gently on the soles of both feet. Allow the heat from your hands to flow into the soles of the receiver's feet. Recommend that the recipient take a deep, slow breath, and you breathe as well. Let your rhythm and the receiver's resonate in a soft, gentle flow of energy.

Hold the right foot, gently moving the foot from side to side; then rotate, changing directions after three turns. Wring the foot from the bottom to the top, and back down again, for three times. You are employing the relaxation techniques as a way to bring all the work together.

Hold the left foot and repeat the gentle movements of turning the foot in and out. Rotate the foot in each direction, turning three times in and then three times out. Wring the foot completely. Bring your hands to the Achilles tendon and the back of the leg, just above the heel. Let one hand cup this area and the other hand firmly hold the top of the foot. The hand holding the top of the foot is wrapped right over the anklebone and is holding gently but firmly.

Imagine the hip, and then with a steady, even yet gentle pressure, pull the leg straight back toward your chest. You will feel a slight answer of pressure flowing back toward you through the leg. As you become aware of this pressure, stop and hold the position. Count to three slowly and release, letting the leg gently relax.

After placing the foot down, move to the right foot and gently cup the heel and hold firmly on the ankle. Again imagine the hip, think of the hip relaxing, and gently pull the leg straight out toward you. Hold once you feel the leg resist, count to three, and release. You'll move on from this to the karate chops. The receiver is aware, on some level, of the transition.

Remember to apply this technique gently. Never pull the leg straight up or too forcefully. This is a loving move that allows complete relaxation of the entire leg and hip. If you do not feel comfortable performing this technique, don't do it.

Karate Chops

The close down can be started on either foot. Most begin on the foot they finished last, which in this case is the left foot. Remember, on the warm-up and cooldown, you have the freedom to move back and forth.

The karate chop technique is first. Hold both hands horizontally to the bottom of the foot; the outside edges of the hands come in contact with the sole. Moving the hands back and forth rapidly, chop from the heel to the toes and back down the foot. Let the fingers of the hands flop loosely against one another. Repeat this chopping motion, up and down the bottom surface, in a steady, rhythmic beat.

> • • • Reflex Points • • •
>
> Although these are called karate chops, you do not use force. Rather, a staccato beat is appropriate. Always work within the receiver's comfort level, using a steady, even tempo. This technique announces to the recipient that you are making a transition, beginning closure.

Karate chops stimulate the feet and the entire body. As you perform this technique you are bringing the receiver's consciousness to the feet. This method relaxes the connective tissue, stimulating the fascia that protects the layers of muscles.

Tapping and Clapping

The tapping technique is another method used in the close-down routine. Steady, rhythmic tapping, with all the fingers, results in a warm feeling on the sole's surface. You may actually see the skin pink up. Using both hands, tap gently and progressively along the surface of the foot, top and bottom. Tap along the sides as well, letting the entire foot feel the sensation.

Use both hands on the foot you are working on. With the foot sandwiched in between the hands, clap. The full hand claps on the foot's surface. The foot feels protected and stimulated. Repeat this on the other foot. You are applauding the feet for receiving the treatment.

Double Solar Plexus Press

Using this powerful technique in closure covers many arenas. Press into both solar plexus reflexes at the same time. Using your fingers, reach up to the toes and gently pull the toe tops down toward the thumb. As the toes pull down, press in further at the reflex.

Ask the receiver to take a slow, deep, and full breath. Remind the receiver to hold the breath for a moment, and then to slowly release it. Encourage the receiver to imagine the breath flowing down the legs and out of the feet. Instruct the receiver to relax and breathe normally.

Press in again, asking the receiver to breathe in slowly, this time attaching her favorite color to the breath. Let the person imagine the breath coming up to the top of her head. You are steadily pressing into the solar plexus reflexes. Now let the receiver slowly release the breath, imagining the color washing down the body and out of the feet. After a second of relaxing, follow this procedure once more.

This process allows the receiver to fully embrace the relaxation. This also encourages the receiver to recognize that the session is ending.

Quiet, Please

The session is complete, the receiver is relaxed, and the music is playing quietly. Adjust the cover on the recipient, making sure she or he is comfortable. Dim the lights or alter the window shades as you leave the room to wash your hands. It is important to allow this quiet moment. All stimuli have been removed; nothing within this energy can create tension. Balance and harmony are restored and remembered. The receiver will keep this stress-free memory, recalling this moment again and again as needed.

••• Reflex Points •••

Do not let the receiver get up immediately. Create an atmosphere that encourages an enjoyable rest time. A progression from total relaxation back to reality must be allowed. Help the receiver to become grounded before leaving the chair. A glass of water, given when the receiver is in an upright position, usually is effective.

Reflexology gives the body, mind, and spirit a feeling of renewal. The receiver is calmer, stronger, and more energized by the treatment. Always include a time of quiet at the end of the session to bring together the substance of the treatment.

After you have washed your hands, it is time to sit the receiver up in the chair. Let the receiver sit for a bit, becoming centered and focused.

Congratulations!

The surprising and delightful plus to this work is the empowerment of the receiver. You have just completed a relaxing and refreshing reflexology session! The person in the chair is better equipped to deal with life's daily stresses than when she or he walked in. The actual reflexing has allowed the receiver to de-stress and recharge. This is a joyful work we do!

The Mini-Session

Many times you will find yourself in situations where the full session may not be appropriate. For example, a younger child may not sit still for an entire session but may benefit from a shorter version. Or, time may be limited, such as at health fairs or community centers.

••• Reflex Points •••

Reflexology mini-sessions work all the zones of the feet, allowing the practitioner to provide a soothing treatment. Comprehensive coverage of all reflexes and points is completed in the longer, full session. By contrast, a shorter version is a successful way to demonstrate the techniques, while also providing a service.

In the Beginning

Always ask the person or the caretaker of the person for information about any key health issues. Ask the potential receiver if she or he has any health concerns that you need to be aware of. People will share their pertinent information when they hear that you genuinely wish to know.

After listening for any current complaints, move on to clean the feet. Disposable sanitary wipes (alcohol- and fragrance-free), the kind used for babies, are a good cleansing tool. While you clean the feet assess for any open cuts or areas that need to be covered, such as plantar warts. Note that there are some instances when a reflexology session may not be appropriate (more on that in the next chapter).

What Is Included

Keep in mind that you should always begin the mini-session with the complete warm-up. Begin on the right foot and use all the warm-up methods, then move to the left foot (see Chapter 7).

Return to the right and thumb walk all the toes, to the edge of the foot and back to the center, once through. Knuckle press the entire bottom of the foot a few times.

Heel press along and thumb walk the sciatic line, then heel press the heel and move on. Thumb walk the zones, and you have finished the right foot. Repeat this process on the left foot, ending with the zones.

Karate chops will announce the end of the session. Notice how relaxed the recipient is. This mini-session does relax and balance the receiver. Once the close-down sequence is complete on both feet, finish the treatment with the double solar plexus press.

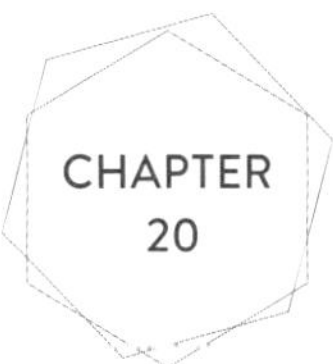

CHAPTER 20

When Is Reflexology Not a Good Idea?

What makes you great is not what you do, but how you do what you do.

—CONSTANCE CHUKS FRIDAY

Although reflexology is quite safe and doesn't harm people, occasionally a referral to a medical practitioner may be appropriate. Certain conditions require medical assistance as well as complementary treatments. It is essential for a reflexologist to know when to work on a person and when not to. Before you start a treatment, discuss the health and well-being of the receiver (see Chapter 5). Then use that information to help create a plan. In this chapter, you'll learn what red flags to look for so that you don't give a session when it might be better not to.

• • • Reflex Points • • •

A reflexologist never tells a receiver what to do with regard to medical treatment. A reflexologist supports and encourages the recipient's journey toward wellness. The receiver's medical doctor will change or adjust the medical treatment as necessary.

No-Go Situations

Under certain circumstances a reflexologist will not even consider working on a person. Here are two you may encounter:

- **Deep vein thrombosis is a blood clot.** If a receiver has this condition, the reflexologist should not work on the feet without a doctor's permission. Often people are treated for this condition with clot-preventing medicines (a detailed receiver history will alert you to this).
- **Compartment syndrome is a condition that is painful and progressive.** Often caused by the repetitive motion of athletic running, this increased pressure and swelling is usually found in the muscles of the lower leg. Pain or loss of feeling in the toes will indicate that this condition is acute! Immediate referral to the emergency room is required.

Make Adjustments

In some cases, an individual with a medical condition can benefit from reflexology as long as some modifications or adjustments to the treatment are made.

Pregnancy

Pregnant women benefit from reflexology, as does the growing baby. The mini-session described in Chapter 19 would be most beneficial during the first three months of pregnancy. Following this, full sessions are acceptable. The professional reflexologist may work through the entire pregnancy, even to being present in the delivery room.

Any bleeding during pregnancy is a cue for immediate referral to the receiver's physician. Many reflexologists find it is best to avoid pressure to the uterus reflex during pregnancy. They may work all other reflexes, which helps to create a warm and loving environment for mother and baby. However, the uterus reflex may be worked during labor.

• • • Reflex Points • • •

Reflexology is very helpful during labor, relaxing the muscles, allowing for increase in circulation, and providing overall relaxation. Of course, permission from the attending caregiver is needed. The laboring mom feels stronger, breathes better, and is more involved when relaxed. Reflexology supports this outcome.

Diabetes

Diabetics benefit from reflexology, as the healing touch encourages peripheral circulation. Diabetes affects the circulation in the body. The supply of blood does not easily reach the nerves in the feet and hands, causing burning pain, unpleasant tingling, even lack of feeling in these extremities. If a reflexologist observes any swelling, cuts, sores, or discoloration in a diabetic receiver's feet, he or she must refer the receiver immediately to the person's medical practitioner.

• • • Reflex Points • • •

Often receivers put off seeking medical attention, not wanting to make a big deal of their condition. Professional reflexologists make it a practice to follow up any suggested referral. They ask the receiver to give an updated report from the medical provider as they offer support and encouragement.

Dilated Varicose Veins

Most varicose veins form pouches that hold the backed-up blood. The veins closer to the skin are more apt to have this weakened condition, which makes the varicose veins visible. Varicose veins are generally bluish in color, at times bulging on the surface of the skin. If a vein is bulging in such a manner, the reflexologist will not finger or thumb walk up the leg. It is best to avoid elevated veins, working the rest of the foot but staying away from these dilated pathways.

Severe Swelling

Swelling of tissue may be caused by kidney or liver dysfunction, a blockage in the circulatory system, or an infection. Any of these conditions would be determined and treated by a medical provider. This swelling may present itself with a pitted surface—as the surface is pressed, it does not spring back. The swelling may be very severe, accompanied by hot or cool temperature, either indicating a systemic condition. Reflexology would not be used under these circumstances unless and until a doctor permitted such treatment.

• • • Reflex Points • • •

Swelling may indicate an internal injury, such as torn ligaments, resulting in a sprain, strain, or fracture. Do not work on an ankle or foot that is swollen and painful. In such cases, immediate referral to the primary care physician is needed.

Some swelling may indicate simple fluid retention. Some people retain fluid because they work on their feet constantly. People who stand all day without much movement may develop chronic swollen ankles. Once a doctor has ruled out any underlying conditions, you can use reflexology in such situations.

Blisters, Open Sores, or Cuts

Any blisters, open sores, or cuts should not be touched, for the health and safety of the receiver as well as the giver. Generally, people have covered these before arriving for the session. If not, keep a supply of good, strong-sticking adhesive bandages on hand.

Be aware that open sores may indicate deeper, underlying, chronic conditions, such as diabetes, or may be related to contagious skin disorders.

Contagious or Infectious Conditions

The feet may have some conditions that a reflexologist should not work on. Athlete's foot is one such condition. Prevention is the best remedy for this condition. Basic healthcare, such as drying feet, especially in between the toes after bathing, is a crucial prevention practice. Keeping the feet as dry as possible is also a preventive measure. Wearing clean, dry white cotton athletic socks helps to prevent the warm environment needed for the growth of this fungus.

Nail Fungus

Nail fungus generally grows in the same environment as athlete's foot. The nail may become thick and raised. A discoloration may appear with some nail fungus. You can work on these nails, though it is good practice to keep disposable gloves in your work area. Use gloves for the first part of the session if the nails are really affected. If gloves were used, remove the gloves before continuing.

• • • Reflex Points • • •

Always make a referral to a medical professional; do not diagnose any condition. Establishing a relationship with a local podiatrist is good practice and will help you better serve those people who do not have a podiatric doctor of their own.

Plantar Warts

Plantar warts may look like a callus, but they are infectious viral conditions of the skin. The center of the wart will have tiny black or red dots and is painful when squeezed from the side. If pushing from the top causes the pain, it is probably a callus or corn. Again, it is not your job to diagnose; leave that to medical professionals. A plantar wart is a virus; therefore, you should cover this spot before working on the feet. Small round adhesive bandages work well as covers. Then you can thumb walk over the area.

Poison Oak, Ivy, and Sumac

Exposure to these plants can cause an allergic contact dermatitis, which may produce itchy, fluid-filled blisters on the body. If a receiver has such blisters on the feet, ankles, or legs, do not work on the area! Explain to the receiver that until the reaction has run its course, the lesions could continue to spread. Recommend the receiver check with his or her physician before returning.

Soft-Tissue Infections

Whenever you have a question relating to your visual assessment of the receiver's feet, it is best to make a referral to a podiatrist. If you find bumps, blisters, scratches, cuts, sores, raw lesions, or any other irregularities that you are not sure of, you need a doctor's okay to work on those areas. Never perform reflexology if you have no knowledge of what is on the person's foot. You do not want to spread infection further, nor do you want exposure through contact.

Current Break or Sprains

A break in a bone may also be called a fracture. A reflexologist does not work on a broken bone until the attending physician gives permission. Reflexology does allow the receiver to relax, assisting in the healing; therefore, you can work on areas of the foot that are not broken (or you can work on the hands).

A sprain occurs when the joint is twisted, such as by an accidental wrenching of the foot. The muscles and connective tissue surrounding the joints become inflamed, and the ligaments that connect the anklebone may swell, become bruised, and even become painful. Application of ice and elevation of the foot is the first response, in conjunction with an immediate referral to a doctor.

Once the doctor has determined that there is no tear in the ligaments, reflexology can help with the swelling and pain. The entire procedure must be gentle, with slow, even movements. Avoid turning, pulling, or chopping methods when a receiver is healing from a sprain.

Fever

Fever is nature's way of indicating something is out of balance within the body. Homeostasis is affected. The cause of a fever could be an infection, either bacterial or viral. However, a fever may come from a heart attack, tumor, surgery, or trauma.

The return of homeostasis is the ideal outcome of a fever. Reflexology can assist in working with the body to speed up this process. Once the cause of the fever has been determined, reflexology can integrate with other modalities, working to create harmony.

APPENDIX A:
REFLEXOLOGY REFERENCE CHARTS

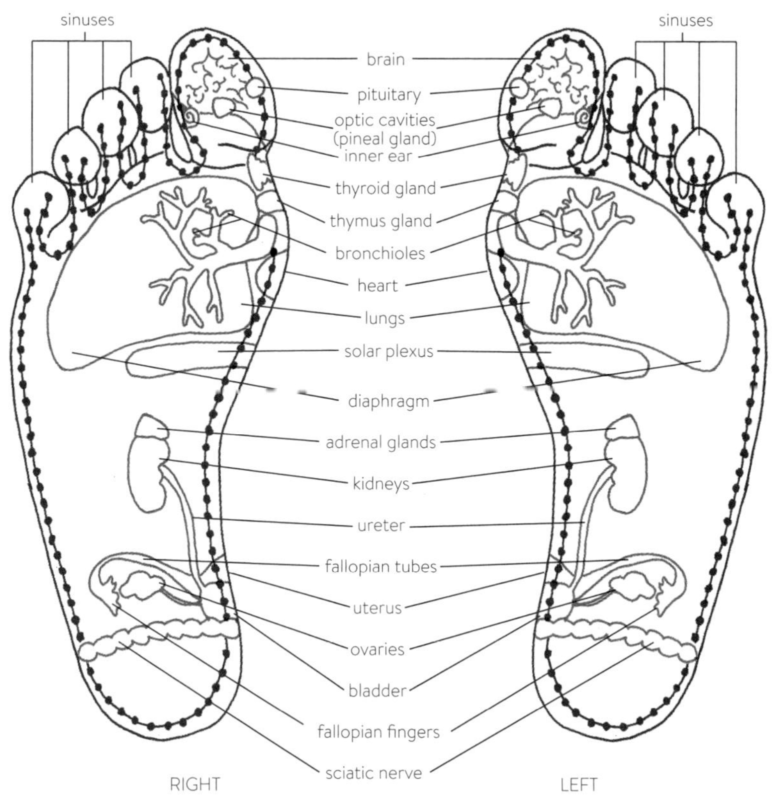

Figure A.1 Foot Chart 1

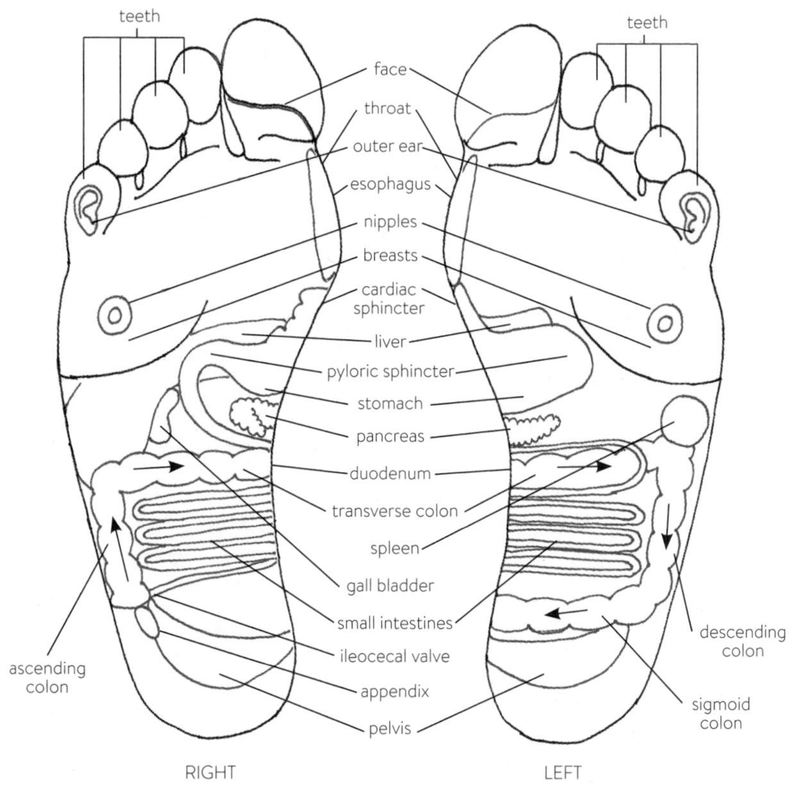

Figure A.2 Foot Chart 2

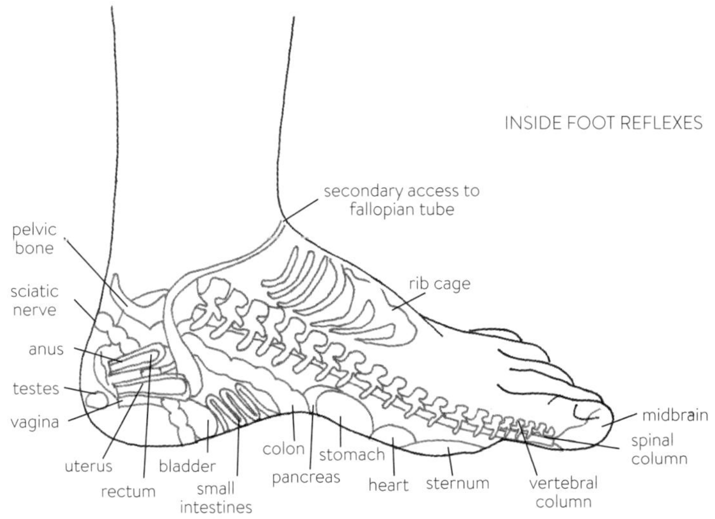

Figure A.3 Inside Foot Chart

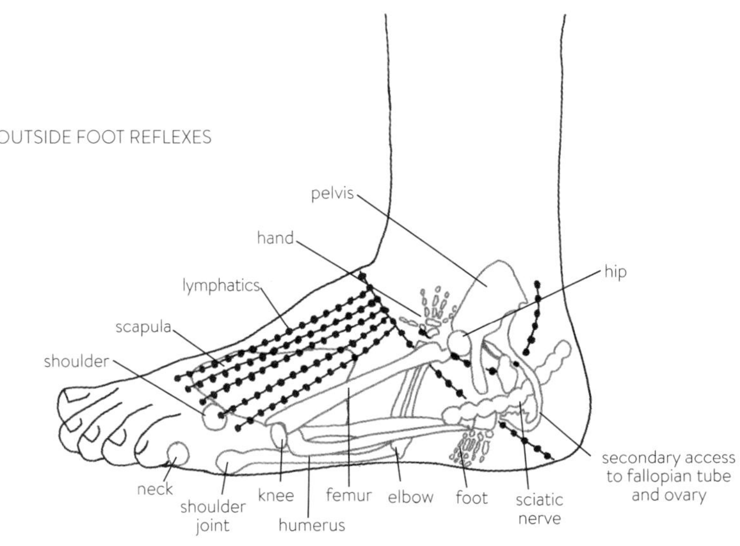

Figure A.4 Outside Foot Chart

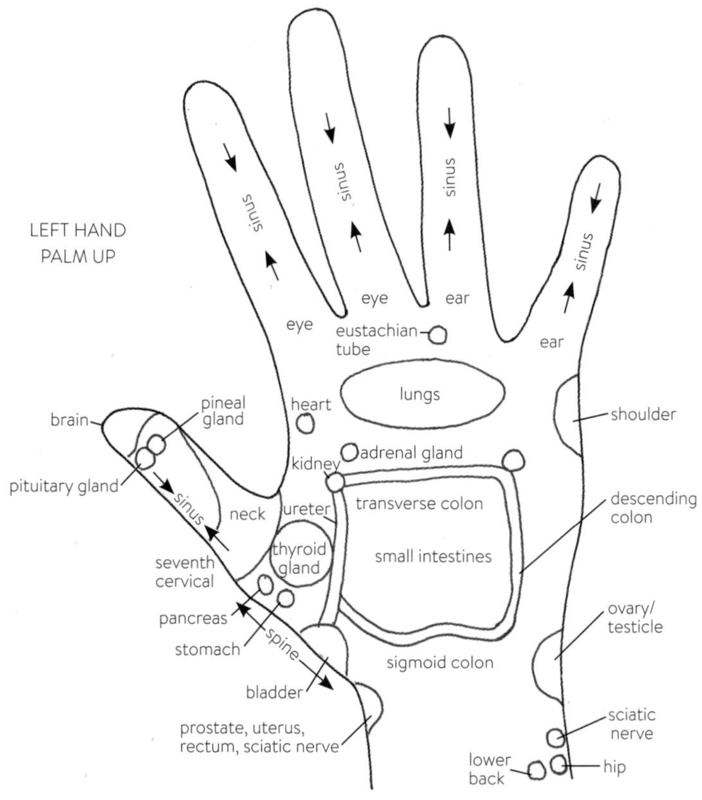

Figure A.5 Hand Chart

APPENDIX B: RESOURCES

Books

Adamson, Suzanne, and Eilish Harris. *The Reflexology Partnership.*

Bayly, Doreen E. *Reflexology Today.*

Berkson, Devaki. *The Foot Book.*

Brown, Denise Whichello. *Reflexology Basics.*

Carter, Mildred, and Tammy Weber. *Body Reflexology.*

Cosway-Hayes, Joan. *Reflexology for Every Body.*

Dougans, Inge. *The Complete Illustrated Guide to Reflexology.*

Gillanders, Ann. *The Busy Person's Guide to Reflexology.*

Hall, Nicola M. *Reflexology.*

Hess, Shelley. *The Professional's Reflexology Handbook.*

Ingham, Eunice D. *Stories the Feet Have Told Thru Reflexology.*

Kaiser, Jürgen, Alexander Scharmann, and Beate Poyck-Scharmann. *Hand Reflexology.*

Kunz, Kevin, and Barbara Kunz. *Hand and Foot Reflexology.*

Manzanares, J. *Principles of Reflexology.*

Marquardt, Hanne. *Reflexotherapy of the Feet.*

Oxenford, Rosalind. *Discover Reflexology.*

Pritt, Donald S., and Morton Walker. *The Complete Foot Book.*

Reid, Elsa, and Susanne Enzer. *Maternity Reflexology.*

Rick, Stephanie. *The Reflexology Workout.*

Rude, Paul. *Souls to Soles.*

Sachs, Judith, and Judith Berger. *Reflexology: The A-Z Guide to Healing with Pressure Points.*

Stormer, Chris. *Teach Yourself Reflexology.*

Vennells, David F. *Reflexology for Beginners.*

Wills, Pauline. *The Reflexology Manual.*

Wolfe, Frankie Avalon. *The Complete Idiot's Guide to Reflexology*.

The American Reflexology Certification Board

The American Reflexology Certification Board (ARCB) is a nonprofit board that offers the voluntary national certification test. ARCB has been and continues to be a standard-setting guideline for the profession of reflexology. Most schools base their curriculum on the requirements established by this board. ARCB in conjunction with the schools has set a continuing-education principle that allows qualified schools and instructors to offer further education in reflexology. Any reflexologist wishing to expand the knowledge of her or his practice will find information through ARCB.

The American Reflexology Certification Board (ARCB)
303-933-6921
www.arcb.net

APPENDIX C:
GLOSSARY

abduction:
The movement of the foot away from the center or midline of the body.

acute:
A condition that is immediate and severe.

adduction:
The movement of the foot toward the center of the body.

allergies:
A hypersensitivity to certain substances that may manifest in negative reactions.

anterior:
The directional term in anatomy that indicates the front of the body.

arches:
We have three arches in the foot; these help to carry weight, absorb shock, and maintain balance.

arthritis:
This painful disease results in inflammation of the joints and affects mobility.

athlete's foot:
The medical terminology is *tinea pedis*, which means "fungus of the foot"; this condition may be caused by fungus or allergic reaction.

back up:
This is part of the reflex technique used when a reflexologist pinpoints a reflex.

biomechanic:
This is the mechanics of movement and balance in dealing with the body.

blisters:
A skin irritation generally caused by rubbing from ill-fitting shoes.

calcaneus:
This is the largest foot bone; it is the heel.

callus:
Hardened layers of skin caused by pressure. The pressure comes from the way we walk or ill-fitting shoes. Generally, calluses are found on the bottom of the foot.

chronic:
A condition that lasts for a long time, showing no improvement, such as chronic pain.

corns:
Calluses found on the top of the foot, on or in between the toes. Corns are usually caused by ill-fitting shoes.

cranial:
This is an anatomical term pertaining to direction. Cranial is near the head, or skull.

cuboid:
A bone of the foot that sits behind the fourth and fifth metatarsal.

cuneiforms:
Bones of the foot that sit behind the first, second, and third metatarsal.

detoxify:
A state when toxins leave the body.

diaphragm line:
The imaginary horizontal line on the foot, denoting the separation of reflexes reflected on the chest and upper abdomen.

distal:
This is a term of direction meaning "away from the point of origin," with the origin being the body.

dislocation:
The displacement of a bone from its joint, with a tearing of ligaments, tendons, and articular capsules.

dorsal:
This is the top of the foot or top of the hand. Dorsal also means the back of the body.

dorsiflexion:
The direction of this movement is bending the foot up toward the body.

eczema:
A condition of the skin, which may cause itching and scaling.

endocrine system:
This system in the body produces the hormones that go directly into the bloodstream.

eversion:
A specific ankle movement that turns the sole of the foot away from the center of the body.

extend:
A movement of muscles that increases range.

fascia:
A connective tissue in the body that provides protection.

flexor:
A movement of muscles causing a bending motion.

fungus:
An infection caused by yeast or mold.

gout:
This form of arthritis is generally found around the first metatarsal head and is caused by an excess of uric acid in the body.

great toe:
One of the anatomical terms used for the big toe.

hallux:
The Latin term for the great toe (big toe).

hallux abducto valgus:
This is the Latin terminology used to describe what is commonly known as a bunion.

hinge joint:
The movement of this joint is like that of a hinged door; generally, the joint is used to flex and extend.

holistic:
This is the body, mind, and spirit concept that reflexology practitioners ascribe to. Healing includes all these parts.

homeostasis:
The anatomical term used to describe the internal balance of the body.

inversion:
This is an ankle movement that turns the sole of the foot in toward the center.

joints of the foot:
The joints of the feet are either hinge joints or gliding joints.

lateral:
The lateral direction is toward the outside of the body.

lateral column:
This area of the foot is used for support.

ligament:
Connective tissue that connects bones to bones.

medial:
This directional term means toward the midline of the body.

medial column:
The inside of the foot used for balance.

metatarsal bones:
These bones connect from the base of the toes to four of the bones of the midfoot.

metatarsophalangeal joint (MTP):
The MTP is the joint that bends the toes up and down.

midline:
Meaning toward the centerline of the body.

muscle:
These are tissues used for motion.

navicular:
This bone connects between the ankle and the three cuneiform bones.

outer longitudinal arch:
This outer arch of the foot carries most of the body's weight.

phalanges:
Anatomical name for the toes.

plantar:
The term used for the bottom of the foot.

plantar fasciitis:
A painful condition on the sole of the foot; it is an inflammation due to strain on the fascia.

plantar flexion:
When the foot is bent down.

plantar wart:
This is a viral infection generally found on the floors of pools, gyms, locker rooms, and public bathing facilities. Its proper name is *verruca plantaris*.

pronation:
This is a movement of the foot involving abduction, eversion, and dorsiflexion.

reflex:
An automatic response to a stimulus. Or, a point on the feet, or hands, that reflects an area of the body.

reflexology:
Applied pressure to reflex points on the hands and feet using specific finger techniques.

sprain:
A forceful trauma to a joint with injury to muscles, ligaments, tendons, and nerves.

spurs:
A buildup of calcium in response to stress in the fascia.

strain:
An overstretching of a muscle.

supination:
This three-plane movement involves adduction, inversion, and plantar flexion.

talus:
This is what is known as the anklebone. Unique to this bone is the fact that there are no muscles attached to it.

tendon:
This is connective tissue that connects muscle to bone.

toenails:
These are protective coverings for the toes.

varicose veins:
A blockage in the veins causing a twisted, ropy, or bumpy protrusion, often on the leg.

weak arches:
Generally, these are fallen arches or commonly known as flatfeet.

yin/yang:
A Chinese concept dealing with balance.

zones:
These are imaginary lines, either vertical or horizontal, that are used as guidelines in reflexology.

INDEX

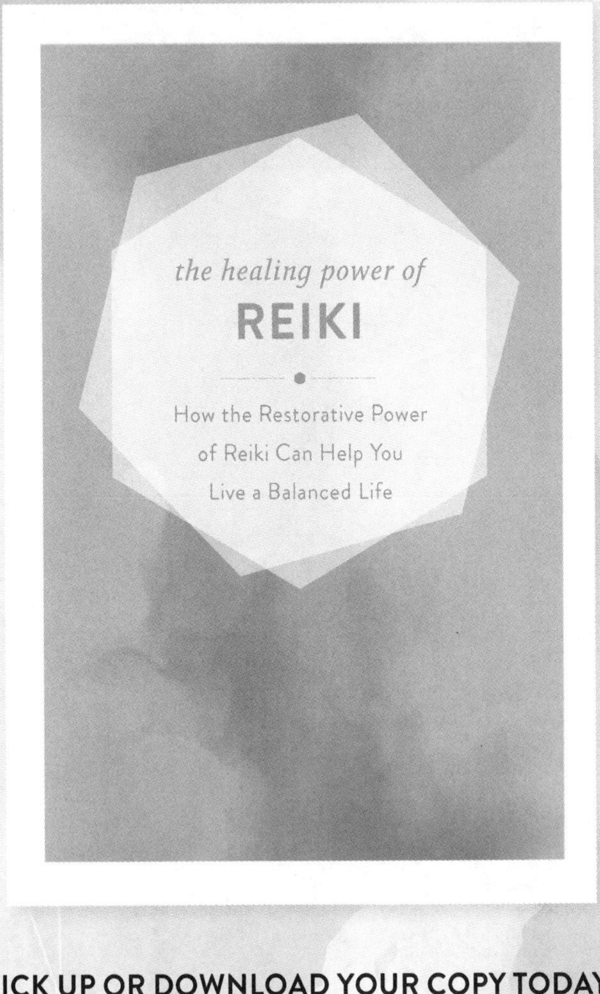